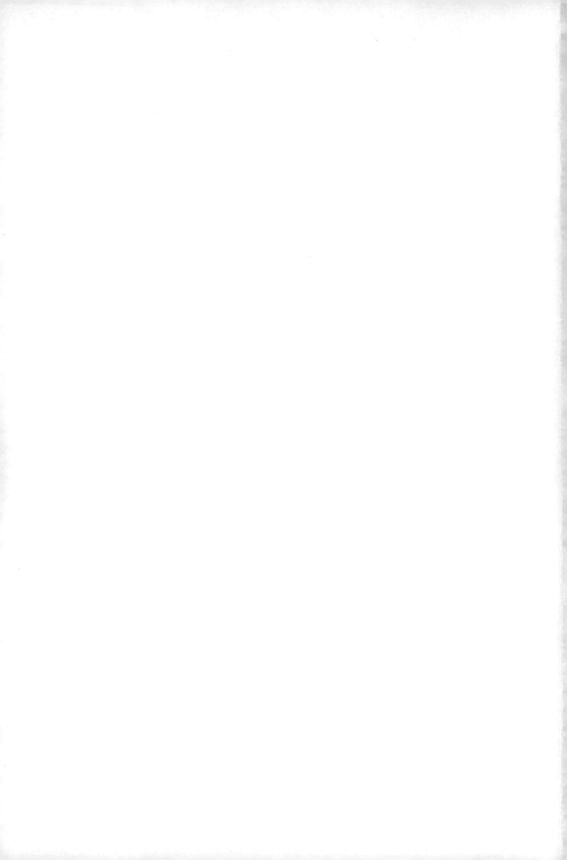

In Her Own Right

The Institute of Medicine's
Guide to Women's Health Issues

By Beryl Lieff Benderly for the Institute of Medicine

NATIONAL ACADEMY PRESS
Washington, D.C. 1997

National Academy Press • 2101 Constitution Avenue, N.W. • Washington, D.C. 20418

NOTICE: The project that is the subject of this report was approved by the Governing Board of the National Research Council, whose members are drawn from the councils of the National Academy of Sciences, the National Academy of Engineering, and the Institute of Medicine.

This report has been reviewed by a group other than the authors according to procedures approved by a Report Review Committee consisting of members of the National Academy of Sciences, the National Academy of Engineering, and the Institute of Medicine.

The Institute of Medicine was chartered in 1970 by the National Academy of Sciences to enlist distinguished members of the appropriate professions in the examination of policy matters pertaining to the health of the public. In this, the Institute acts under the Academy's 1863 congressional charter responsibility to be an adviser to the federal government and its own initiative in identifying issues of medical care, research, and education. Dr. Kenneth I. Shine is president of the Institute of Medicine.

This project was supported in part by a grant from the Johnson & Johnson Family of Companies.

Printed in the United States of America

Cover: Madge Tennent. *Local Color*, 1934. Oil on canvas. The National Museum of Women in the Arts. On loan from the Tennent Art Foundation.

The serpent has been a symbol of long life, healing, and knowledge among almost all cultures and religions since the beginning of recorded history. The image adopted as a logo-type by the Institute of Medicine is based on a relief carving from ancient Greece, now held by the Staatlichemuseen in Berlin.

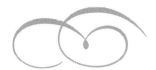

Contents

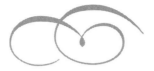

Acknowledgments

The Institute of Medicine acknowledges with gratitude the contributions of the many people who have lent their efforts and expertise to this project during its planning and inception, writing, and production. Among these people are the speakers at the Institute's 1992 annual meeting and the 1991 Symposium on Nutrition, Women, and Their Health; the author, Beryl Lieff Benderly, who organized and made more accessible a vast amount of material; the editor, Roseanne Price, who helped refine the text; past and present Institute staff, including Enriqueta Bond, under whose stewardship as executive officer the project was conceived and largely executed; Karen Hein, IOM's current executive officer, who has seen it to its completion; and Judith Auerbach, Sue Barron, Conrad Baugh, Claudia Carl, Lou Cranford, Michael Edington, Polly Harrison, Chris Howson, Sandra Matthews, Patty Olender, Janet Stoll, Carol Suitor, Paul Thomas, Betsy Turvene, Catherine Woteki, and Allison Yates; and the staff at the National Academy Press—Dawn Eichenlaub, Barbara Kline Pope, Estelle Miller, Francesca Moghari, Brooke O'Donnell, and Sally Stanfield—who have applied their art and craft to the book's design and publication. All of these people have helped to shape the volume you now hold in your hands. Finally, the Institute is especially grateful to the Johnson & Johnson Family of Companies for the financial support that made this project a reality.

In Her Own Right

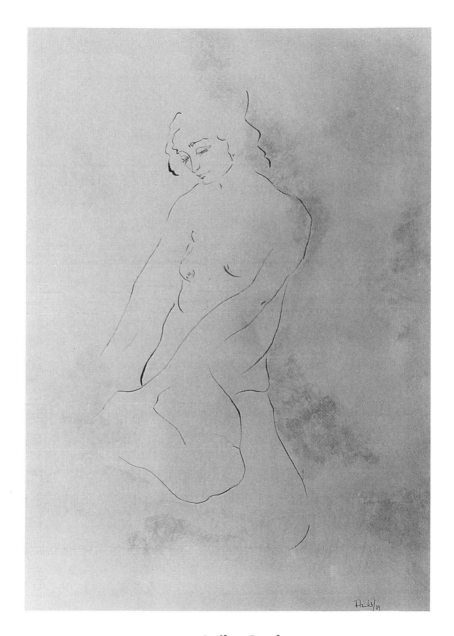

Aniko Gaal
Meditation (1979)
Watercolor and ink on paper
The National Museum of Women in the Arts
Gift of Wallace and Wilhelmina Holladay

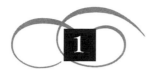

Why Another Book on Women's Health?

A large headline scowls from the front page of a metropolitan daily. Below it, a grainy photo captures a middle-aged man frowning over his bifocals. EXPERTS QUESTION SAFETY OF MAJOR BREAST CANCER STUDY, the heavy type proclaims. A line of smaller print identifies the man, a medical school professor, as a "leading critic of the tamoxifen trial."

A blond movie actress beams at an even blonder toddler on an eye-level rack above a supermarket checkout counter. Over her head marches the bright-red name of a national women's magazine. Next to her, lines of variegated type promise a late bulletin about the Kennedy family, announce the advent of a surefire weight loss plan, and pose a pair of disquieting queries: WHAT TO DO ABOUT MENOPAUSE? IS HORMONE THERAPY FOR YOU?

I ssues involving women's health are everywhere these days. Questions once discussed only in the privacy of the consulting room, matters formerly considered either too personal or too technical for general conversation, decisions that used to be left to experts, now pop up across kitchen tables, in parking lots, and over office coffee machines across the nation. How much the nation spends on what kinds of medical research, once an esoteric interest of academics, now inspires protest marches. Concern about reproductive diseases, once whispered among close friends, now finds expression in bits of ribbon pinned to lapels.

The last decades have seen a truly startling change. From the specialized concerns of a small number of activists, clinicians, and scholars, women's health issues have grown into a major preoccupation of political leaders, medical researchers, and the popular media. The first edition of the now-perennial bestseller, *Our Bodies, Ourselves,* constituted a daring departure from accepted thinking. A White House announcement that the First Lady faced breast cancer surgery created a national sensation, linking the President's family to the then-unprintable words "breast" and "cancer."

A new generation of women began to develop a new sense of themselves as consumers of health care services. And the unprecedented official candor about Betty Ford's and, soon afterward, Second Lady Happy Rockefeller's, mastectomies made the subject instantly respectable, sent millions of women to seek mammograms, and sparked reformers to begin questioning the disfiguring orthodoxy of total breast removal.

Today, as female physicians stream out of medical schools and residency programs in record numbers, health issues important to women have moved—along with other formerly ignored issues like family leave and pay inequities—to the forefront of national consciousness. Major dailies now headline developments in diseases once considered unfit for mention in family newspapers. Women's magazines delve into the choices open to informed health care consumers. Television newscasts highlight controversial research results. Bookstore shelves overflow with volumes on every aspect of the female mind and body. Videos, tapes, newsletters, computer bulletin boards, and every other available mode of communication constantly add to the rising torrent of information, guidance, and opinion.

So why should the Institute of Medicine (IOM), a scientific body chartered by the U.S. Congress to provide expert consultation on pressing public issues, enter so crowded a field? Why should an organization customarily devoted to detailed consideration of technical matters give a popular treatment to an already over-covered topic? And perhaps most significantly for the reader, why add yet another voice to the din?

The most pressing reason is that din is exactly what all too often answers a thoughtful citizen's efforts to stay informed. As authors of particular books, advocates for selected diseases, and proponents of various theories compete on talk shows and in op-ed pieces and magazine articles for viewers' and readers' limited attention, no sense of priority or relative importance orders the discussion. Every disease appears equally dreadful, every threat equally dire, every risk equally grave. In the new world of health awareness, however, ordinary citizens are no longer patients shepherded by fatherly medical advisors but consumers of services and information in a competitive marketplace. Confronted with any important medical problem, ordinary people are increasingly encouraged, even required, to make the kind of decisions once the exclusive province of doctors.

In this new atmosphere, understanding how to frame intelligent questions has become surpassingly important. What are the risks and benefits of various forms of birth control? What are the health costs of delaying childbearing—or of proceeding with it too early? Should a meno pausal woman take hormone replacement therapy? And if so, for how long? Should a breast cancer patient opt for lumpectomy or mastectomy? For post-surgical medication? Issues like these—real, serious questions with real, serious, though not necessarily knowable, consequences—face more and more people in our age of informed consent and increasingly impersonal care. Where once those without medical training left such matters in the hands of a trusted adviser who knew us personally and took a paternalistic interest in our welfare, today, professionals increasingly expect lay people, frequently under extreme emotional stress, to quickly learn enough gynecology or oncology or cardiology to participate in the deliberations and make the final choices among available options.

In this new age, then, anyone who has ever been or expects to be a patient, or who has ever had or expects to have responsibility for the health care of others, needs a framework to organize what they know, to give fragments of information the meaning and priority only possible as parts of a systematic body of understanding.

Clearly, no untrained person can expect to acquire, nor can any popular book claim to deliver, the detailed, comprehensive grasp that a health professional has. But high-level expertise is not what best serves today's intelligent health care consumer. Rather, she or he needs a way of thinking about medical information, a way of sorting out claims and weighing results. How, for example, does one know if a drug is "safe" (considering that all medications have side effects and taking any at all constitutes a bet on expected benefits over possible harm)? What are the major health threats a woman should take care to guard against (considering that, contrary to popular impression, heart disease kills many more females than breast cancer)? What is the best way to counter obesity (remembering that some weight loss methods in themselves represent threats to health)? Providing a framework for thinking about such issues is what this book aims to do.

Two circumstances spurred this effort, one relating to the subject itself, the other to the nature of the IOM. Many of the topics that flash across the national consciousness and briefly flood the popular media are fads or frivolities. The current interest in women's health clearly is not. A number of the changes in thinking taking place not only among the general public but also among health professionals represent, at their intellectual base, a thoroughgoing and long overdue reassessment.

The medical enterprise, both in scientific research and in clinical practice has traditionally viewed female lives and bodies through a lens of masculine experience and assumptions. Indeed, the name of the medical specialty that studies female reproduction, gynecology, means "science of woman" in Greek. No corresponding specialty of "andrology" studies the distinctive reproductive features of men. Male reproduction falls instead under urology, literally, "the science of urine," which, according to a leading medical dictionary, encompasses "the study, diagnosis and treatment of diseases of the genitourinary tract, especially the urinary tract in both sexes and the genital organs in the male."[1] Male genitalia, in other words, form a subdivision of a larger, more general, bodily system, while female reproductive organs occupy a special realm, distinct from the body at large, and one that also just happens to define their owner's essential nature.

The effort to remove this distorting lens, to see and treat the female person as a whole and normal human being in her own right, rather than as a subsidiary or deviant version of the dominant male, is already well under way. The need to incorporate female experience and perceptions into medical thinking has become obvious across the health care community.

Informing the public of the issues at stake is basic to this effort of reexamination and reform. Realigning a field of knowledge, reformulating an area of endeavor, requires a new architecture for thought and analysis. In the famous phrase of the historian of science Thomas Kuhn, it requires a "paradigm shift." Scholars and scientists have already begun sketching out a new paradigm for women's health, a new image of the physical and mental well-being of half the human race. To show how this new thinking applies to the lives of real people of both genders is the goal of this book.

The Institute of Medicine brings to this effort two special resources, the breadth of its exposure to health issues and the depth of its expertise. Throughout its history, IOM has assembled committees of recognized experts to study major health issues and has organized meetings to present the latest and most authoritative views in fast-moving research fields. A quarter-century of unbiased study and consensual decision making, besides creating a large body of trustworthy information, offers protection from the vagaries of fashion and the extremes of ideology. In the changing world of women's health, as with many other major social changes, important and sometimes well-financed interests have lined up on various sides of various questions. In its many studies and meetings, IOM has striven for fair, balanced, and responsible consideration.

A subject long central to the Institute's work has now moved to the center of the nation's attention. Concerns specific to women—reproductive technology, breast cancer, osteoporosis, menopause—now receive wide coverage. Issues shared with men but predominantly affecting women—aging, depression, obesity, sexual harassment, child care—increasingly dominate the news. Newly salient policy questions, like the design of clinical trials, crop up in the popular media.

Symbolizing and enhancing the new prominence of women's concerns, the Institute and its constituent body, the Food and Nutrition Board, have explored them in a variety of publications and at two major conferences. In December 1991, FNB examined nutrition and its effect on women's health. In October 1992, IOM used its annual meeting to take stock of gender as it relates to health and health care. Covered in both professional and popular media, these gatherings focused attention on factors that crucially affect the physical and mental well-being of women and girls around the world. Though the meetings involved different scholarly bodies and emphasized different scientific disciplines, both sought answers to the same central questions: Which factors contribute to—or detract from—women's mental and physical well-being? How can that well-being be improved? What accounts for discrepancies in the health of men and women? How can inequities be corrected?

Or, as a Food and Nutrition Board conference speaker, Susan Scrimshaw, Ph.D., professor and associate dean at the UCLA School of Public Health,★ put it most succinctly, the question comes down to "Why women?" Why do the things that happen specifically to women happen to them and not to men? Why do they face numerous health risks much rarer among men—breast cancer, eating disorders, high rates of anemia and depression, to name just a few? What is it about their lives that opens them to these problems? How can those conditions be improved?

Three themes that form the leitmotifs of IOM work lead the way toward answers: different biologies and physiologies, divergent life courses, and unequal social statuses. Males and females have bodies that differ in important respects. They still have remarkably dissimilar experiences in growing up, during maturity, and as they age. And, despite the rapid social change of the last generation, they still play different roles in society and face different pressures and expectations.

No one of these factors in itself completely explains such puzzles as women's higher morbidity but lower mortality, their greater susceptibility to depression, or the inadequate nourishment they receive in many parts of the world. Clearly, differences in the genders' patterns of health and illness arise both from physical factors like women's more responsive immune systems and from social factors like their greater exposure to children and the sick. The health care system also treats the genders differently, for example, in its approach to cardiac illness.

Dietary differences also carry important consequences. Common conditions like anemia and osteoporosis arise from a combination of dietary and behavioral causes. The former occurs often among poorly nourished but frequently pregnant women, and the latter among those who consumed too little calcium in their youth and got too little exercise in maturity. A similar combination of food and lifestyle—specifically, high fat and late childbearing—is heavily implicated in the industrialized West-

---

★The affiliations cited for the speakers throughout this volume have not been updated—ED.

ern countries' high rates of breast cancer. Along with their special social roles, women clearly face distinctive nutritional challenges, especially when the heavy demands of childbirth and nursing come on top of general requirements for good health.

But beyond those uniquely feminine processes, a constellation of physiological and social factors conspires to threaten women's welfare. Many cultures erect specific obstacles that prevent females from eating adequately, barriers not equally applicable to males. In developing countries, most women do heavy labor and endure repeated, closely spaced pregnancies but have less chance than men and children to eat what they need. In the developed world the ideal of slenderness takes hold before adolescence and persists into middle age and beyond, pressing in most severely during the very same adolescent and early adult years when a woman must lay down in her bones a supply of calcium to last her lifetime and when she conceives and bears her children. And in the United States the increasingly parlous state of young women—a confusion of life goals compounded by increasing sexual pressure—has brought on a growing rash of depression, addiction, and eating disorders. Each of these situations merits asking "Why women?" Each affords clues to the realities shaping female lives.

From cases like these and from IOM's work on women's health emerge three overarching themes that form this book's intellectual framework.

Health is the intersection of an individual's physical endowment and life experience. Except in very rare cases, no single factor determines the state of an individual's physical or mental health. Rather, physiology, diet, developmental history, emotional and intellectual experience, social opportunities, physical environment, and other elements all enter the equation.

A woman's health evolves across her entire life span. This statement deserves special note because, surprisingly enough, it represents a departure from the traditional view of the female, which centered on childbearing. Women's reproductive capacity has long formed a major focus of attention. Improving or controlling the ability to bear healthy babies has been the goal of much scientific and clinical work. The study of women's health has often paid more attention to the health of a woman's children than to the mother herself and devoted more resources to improving their welfare than hers. In much of the developing world, it has focused on childbirth and lactation with little concern for the decades before and after.

Central to the new woman-centered notion of women's health, however, and to this book, is the understanding that women's health concerns deserve to be addressed *as they affect women,* persons who have lives before and after the possibility of childbearing and whose well-being matters whether or not they ever bear children. As is also true for men, health status at every stage of life affects the stages that follow, often in complex, subtle, and unexpected ways. As more and more women live to older and older ages, the total shape of the female life span, of which reproduction constitutes only a limited period, must come into clearer view.

"In 1988 . . . [the] articulation of a 'life-cycle' approach to thinking about female health was novel and innovative," observes a ground-breaking report of IOM's Committee to Study Female Morbidity and Mortality in Sub-Saharan Africa.[2] This perspective assumes the need to articulate the major causes of health status not solely in women of reproductive age, but in "an individual's entire life experience from birth to death, whether or not that includes reproduction."[3]

Women's life experiences and social roles differ from men's in ways that affect physical and mental health. These differences bear heavily on many aspects of health, including such diverse issues as what and how much a woman eats, how and where she gets medical care, and whether the factors affecting her health get appropriate attention in research.

Through its leadership role in medicine, IOM has over the years accumulated a large body of information and insight that illuminates many of the issues surrounding women's health today and tomorrow. This book endeavors to use that resource—specifically, the findings of a variety of reports and conferences—to explain what women (and men) need to know.

NOTES

1. *Stedman's Medical Dictionary*, 25th ed., s.v. "urology."
2. *In Her Lifetime: Female Morbidity and Mortality in Sub-Saharan Africa*, 2.
3. Ibid, 3.

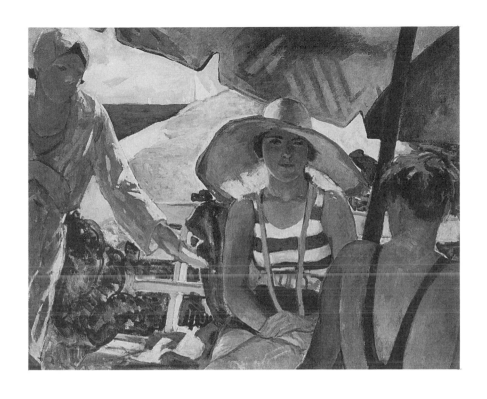

Beatrice Whitney Van Ness
Summer Sunlight (ca. 1936)
Oil on canvas
The National Museum of Women in the Arts
Gift of Wallace and Wilhelmina Holladay

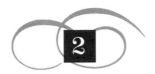

Gender Differences in Health

Both likenesses and differences go back to the very moment of conception. Gender begins in an individual's genes. Of the 46 chromosomes that compose the human genome, 45 distinguish not at all between males and females. The crucial forty-sixth alone determines genetic gender at the moment that sperm meets egg.

In all cells but the type involved in fertilization, chromosomes come two by two, forming a total of 23 pairs. At conception, each parent bestows on each offspring one randomly chosen member of each of his or her pairs. All but one of these pairs consist of two chromosomes equal in size. The gender-picking set, however, comes in two versions, the full-sized X and the much smaller Y. Females possess two Xs, so a mother can only pass along one of that type. Males, however, possess both an X and a Y, so a father can transmit either one.

Each of the father's sperm and each of the mother's eggs, alone of all the cells in the body, contain only 23 individual chromosomes, one from each pair. The process that creates these special cells assigns each individual egg or sperm its particular complement of chromosomes apparently at random. The sperm, in their multitudes, race toward the solitary ovum, each bearing a gender-determining X or Y. One and only one sperm cell penetrates the large, slow-moving prize. At that instant, as the two half-sets of chromosomes combine, the newly formed person-to-be comes into possession of the full genetic complement that will last—and shape—a lifetime. An embryo that happens to receive the paternal Y will almost certainly emerge nine months later to cries of "It's a boy!" One getting two Xs will proceed to develop as a girl.

As a girl, not *into* a girl. In *Homo sapiens*, as in all mammals, the female is the so-called "default" gender; every embryonic human would develop the body of a female if nothing intervened. Early in its growth, each embryo develops two sets of rudimentary ducts, the basic where-withal needed to grow into a mature member of either sex. The müllerian duct stands poised to become uterus and fallopian tubes, the Wolffian, the male reproductive organs. In addition, the embryo's equipment includes as-yet undifferentiated gonadal cells, forerunner of its future ovaries or testes. If specific male-making events do not happen early enough in the pregnancy to derail the process, the müllerian duct grows into full-fledged female organs and the Wolffian duct withers. The thing that permits—indeed, forces—masculine development arrives on the Y chromosome. At the proper developmental moment, before a mother-to-be may even know for sure she is pregnant, the future male's gonads receive a signal to grow into testes. Without this signal, the gonads mature into ovaries.

The Y chromosome thus throws a binary switch that selects between two gender possibilities. But this initial differentiation constitutes only the first, though absolutely crucial, step in the multistage procedure that will result in a male. In engineering parlance, this first step starts a "cascade" of events that broaden its effect far beyond its initial power.

In the second step the newly functioning testes begin producing a substance that directs the müllerian duct to degenerate, erasing the embryo's female potential. Later on, testicular hormones called androgens (literally, "male makers") prod the Wolffian tract to mature, setting out the masculine organs. Unless both these signals reach their destinations, the turn toward masculinity simply does not occur, or occurs incompletely. In such cases, female development proceeds. The rare XY individual whose cells are genetically unable to respond to certain androgens, for example, has the outer appearance, but not the full inner equipment, of a female.

Further along in fetal development, androgens signal the brain to prepare for the time, lying more than a decade in the future, when it will act in a mature male-like way. Specifically, this step lays the ground-work for a masculine rather than a feminine puberty. It assures that the young brain will fail to produce the hormonal feedback loop that orchestrates the menstrual cycle. With the onset of puberty, additional hormones will signal the development of such secondary masculine traits as body hair, the voice-lowering enlargement of the larynx, and the broad shoulders that produce the male rather than the female silhouette.

Within these two distinctly shaped frames, however, many of the infinitely complex mechanisms that compose the human body nonetheless function quite similarly. The doings of chromosome number 46 have riveted society's attention since time immemorial, but the other 45 clearly exert far greater combined influence. Males and females of the human species share an overwhelming number of features of anatomy, physiology, and behavior. Only the organs specifically related to reproduction belong exclusively to one gender or the other. Even secondary sexual characteristics like the female breast and the deeper male voice derive from structures shared by both genders.

These two similar bodies, however, still contain sufficient discrepancies, or perhaps undergo sufficiently different stresses during their lifetimes, to produce quite noticeably discrepant patterns of illness and health. Some differences arise from reasons so obvious as to be trivial; men cannot suffer preeclampsia of pregnancy nor women contract prostate cancer (although men can and do develop breast cancer). More serious and substantive variations—different rates of mental disorder, different ages for heart disease—have spurred spirited debate but as yet inadequate research. Anecdotal evidence from both the bedside and the laboratory suggests still further differences as yet suspected but not definitely proven.

MATTERS OF LIFE AND DEATH

The simplest and most straightforward difference is also the most mysterious. Throughout the developed world, wherever women no longer routinely die in childbirth, women on average live longer than men—6.9 years longer in the United States, for example.[1] Demographers noticed this longevity gap as long ago as 1900, decades before cigarette smoking, once a predominantly male habit, and a major killer of American men for at least 40 years, became commonplace. "It appears to be present in all races and under all social conditions," notes Maureen M. Henderson, M.D., D.P.H., professor of epidemiology and medicine at the University of Washington and a leading expert in the epidemiology of disease.[2]

Nor do the factors favoring females seem to cluster in any particular stretch of the human life span. "Women's survival advantage exists in infancy and childhood, that is, before puberty and circulating levels of reproductive hormones," says Henderson.[3] "At all ages, from conception on," adds Leon E. Rosenberg, M.D., president of the Bristol-Myers Squibb Pharmaceutical Research Institute, relatively more males than females die. "Approximately 125 male fetuses are conceived for every 100 female fetuses, but 27 percent more boys than girls die in the first year of life. By the time they have lived 100 years, women outnumber men five to one."[4] Differentials as marked as these powerfully shape demographics. Women constitute almost 60% of Americans over 65 and 75% of those over 85—the fastest-growing segment of our population.[5]

Exactly what kills the genders at such different rates remains much less obvious. Clearly, both biological and behavioral factors come into play. "One very critical biological component," Henderson suggests, is females' "more responsive immune system." Testing of the hepatitis B vaccine confirmed clinicians' long-standing suspicion that women fight off infectious invaders better than men. "At every age, exposure for exposure, females have better antibody responses."[6] Whether facing bacteria in hospital nurseries, the viruses coughed and sneezed among infants and children, or even, as some suggest, the viruses associated with certain cancers, female immune systems appear to put up stiffer resistance.

But, Henderson acknowledges, "other components of this better female survival have yet to be thoroughly explored and described." Women's recent mass exodus from home to the workplace, for example, has produced no noticeable effect on their death rates, despite predictions that job stresses would push them closer to the pattern of male mortality. But, one factor, she notes, "is slowly and surely lowering women's survival rates closer to men's"—the recent, sharp increase in females smoking cigarettes, particularly among teenage girls and young women. "On balance, however, women are currently holding onto their survival advantage."[7] That fact suggests to some that, given the damage from increased smoking, joining the paid workforce might somehow help rather than harm women's health.

But that mystery only deepens another one. Women, Rosenberg puzzles, "are sicker, but live longer." They spend more days confined to bed, take more time off from work, go to the hospital more, and see doctors more often. No one knows why, but social reasons strike many as likely. How people perceive symptoms, what they think they should do about them, and where they stand in the social structure all influence whether they consider themselves sick. Denying illness, Rosenberg notes, is "culturally approved" behavior that discourages men from seeing a doctor in the first place or complying with instructions when they do.[8]

Cultural factors aside, does the first mystery, women's longer survival, even more paradoxically suggest an answer to the second, their higher disease rate? By living longer, many more of them reach the age range most afflicted by disease. Fewer men make it into old age, so the select number who do may have enjoyed some lifelong advantage in resisting disease. "Men over 75 are a particularly robust group if they manage to survive their cohort, and represent biologically a different group of people than their feminine counterparts," suggests Dr. Bertram Cohler, professor of psychology at the University of Chicago.[9] This smaller and presumably more exclusive group has already lost many young and middle-aged members to some of the very diseases that afflict elderly women. Coronary heart disease, for example, begins taking its toll of males a decade before it attacks females; myocardial infarction strikes men fully two decades earlier than women.[10]

Still, when heart disease finally does attack women, it exacts heavy losses. Women die more often than men do from infarctions and surgeries like bypasses and angioplasties. Does something inherent in women's physiology or anatomy—smaller, more easily blocked blood vessels, for example—account for the difference or discrepancies in diagnosis and treatment? Both possibilities have expert support. Heart conditions often present somewhat differently in women than in men, who, because they were long considered the likeliest victims, have shaped the disease's predominant image. Womens' chest complaints may get more cursory scrutiny, some believe. Indeed, Nanette K. Wenger, M.D., professor of medicine and cardiology at Emory University Medical School, expresses "concern that later diagnosis and less attention to the symptoms" mean that women often miss getting attention during the disease's more treatable early stages and thus need more emergency surgery in the more dangerous late ones. For "both genders and at all ages [such an operation] carries a higher risk of mortality" than one conducted on a nonemergency basis.[11]

The more-selective-male-cohort theory also fails to satisfy some observers. Henderson, for example, sees older women's higher rate of reported disease as simply that, a higher rate of reporting. An ailment swells disease statistics only if and when it comes to a professional's attention. "Women don't suffer from unique conditions"; she notes, "they just report more of the same conditions reported by men."[12] Do they really get sicker more often or do they simply seek care more often when they do? Existing figures, obviously, cannot give the answer.

"Throughout their reproductive and later lives," Henderson continues, underlining Rosenberg's point, "women go to the doctor's office more often than men," a habit that can grow in the early years from needing the most effective forms of birth control, available only by prescription, and in the later ones from seeking annual Pap smears. Once in the doctor's office, a woman usually answers questions about her general health, and may even fill out a checklist, perhaps prompting her to remember or recognize symptoms that in themselves would not merit a special call or visit. When healthy men filled out similar lists in one study, Henderson notes, more of them indicated complaints than a comparable group of women. And, she further wonders, might women's more frequent contact with health professionals "itself lead to treatments whose existence, consequences, and side effects are then reported as symptoms"[?][13]

This possibility certainly exists because elderly women annually consume one-fifth more medication than men—an average of 5.7 prescriptions a year, plus 3.2 different types of over-the-counter remedies. One of every four women over 65 uses 21 different medications annually; only one older man in five uses that many.[14] With overmedication and drug interactions a recognized cause of symptoms in seniors, women are obviously at somewhat greater risk.

The conditions that men and women hope to counter with all these drugs differ by gender as well. Three times as many women as men develop rheumatoid arthritis—possibly a manifestation of that extraactive immune system mistakenly turning on one's own tissues. Men suffer more hearing loss, possibly because they have been exposed to more industrial noise. Osteoporosis, which thins the bones and causes painful and disabling fractures, strikes vastly more often in women, afflicting 73% of those between 65 and 69 and 89% of those over 75.[15] An American woman faces a risk of life-shortening hip fracture three times greater than a man's and as great—15% during her lifetime—as her *combined* total risk of breast, uterine, and ovarian cancer or a man's lifetime risk of prostate cancer. Half of hip fracture victims never walk again, many falling prey to such complications of immobility as pressure sores, urinary infections, heart arrhythmias, and pneumonia. Overall, hip fractures reduce expected survival by 5 to 20%.[16]

So great, in fact, is women's burden of illness and disability in old age that they confront the "horrible travesty" of "not so much living longer, but taking longer to die," in Henderson's words. The grim realities of disease, disability, and resulting loss of independence whittle "their extra seven years of life expectancy . . . down to three good years and four bad."[17]

Men who survive to old age spend a greater proportion of their remaining years free of disability. A man still living independently at 70, for example, can look forward, on average, to another 11.4 years, all but 18% of them still independent. But at 70 an independent woman stands to spend 29% of her remaining 15.4 years in a state of dependency.[18] This gives her only 1.6 more independent years than a man but 2.4 more dependent years. Between 1970 and 1987, women's life expectancy rose 3.6 years, but 3.3 of those years entail some limitation on activities. Men, on the other hand, gained only 2.8 years of life expectancy, but two-thirds of it without limitations.[19]

But since women's greater disease rate persists throughout the life span, age alone cannot explain it. When investigators seek specific diseases to account for the excess, "some of the differences in reported rates of acute infectious conditions during early adult life are logical," Henderson notes, given women's closer contact with youngsters carrying home infections from school and day care and their greater responsibility for all family members who take sick. Probably reflecting a drop in home nursing duties as children mature, "men's and women's reported rates of acute infections get much more alike as they get older."[20]

The same younger women, of an age to be caring for infected small children, are also at the age of highest risk for autoimmune diseases. Might not that more responsive immune system, rallied by the more frequent need to fight infections, sometimes go awry from overenthusiasm? Though these ailments alone do not occur often enough to explain the genders' different illness rates, this is only one of the many questions that await further research.

MIND AND MATTER

More than immune responses and rates of physical illness distinguish male and female health. The realm of mental health involves discrepancies as large or larger. Overall, mental disorders affect about the same proportion of each sex—according to the Epidemiological Catchment Area study of the National Institute of Mental Health, a survey of 18,000 American adults living in five communities—but in strikingly disparate patterns.[21]

A woman is a third again as likely as a man to suffer obsessive-compulsive and bipolar disorders (manic-depression) at some time in her life, one-half again as likely to develop schizophrenia, and twice as likely to suffer phobias (see Table 2-1). She also runs more than twice his risk of panic disorder, major depression, and dysthymia (chronic depression), and seven times his risk of somatization disorder, which involves various bodily symptoms. He, meanwhile, has almost twice the chance she does of abusing drugs, and about five times her chance of abusing alcohol or developing antisocial personality disorder.[22]

Whether gender differences in rates of substance abuse are truly as large as the statistics suggest or whether the discrepancies represent women's hesitancy about coming forward for treatment remains unclear, however. Drunkenness has traditionally carried a greater stigma for fe-

TABLE 2-1 Mental and Addictive Disorders in Women and Men

Disorder	Male Lifetime Rate per 100	Female Lifetime Rate per 100	Odds Ratio
Somatization	0.0002	0.4	7.34
Major depression	2.7	5.7	2.41
Panic disorder	0.8	1.8	2.31
Dysthymia	1.9	3.9	2.06
Phobias	9.5	18.3	1.98
Schizophrenia	1.0	1.6	1.48
Obsessive–compulsive disorder	1.8	2.4	1.33
Bipolar disorder	0.6	0.8	1.29
Drug abuse	6.2	3.7	0.64
Antisocial personality	3.7	0.8	0.18
Alcohol abuse	21.2	4.3	0.15

NOTE: Odds ratios are adjusted for age and socioeconomic status.

SOURCE: Institute of Medicine, *Asssessing Future Research Needs: Mental and Addictive Disorders in Women (Summary)*, 1991.

males than for males. For him, it can indicate toughness, a macho, devil-may-care attitude—up to a point, at least. For her, it often still carries an implication of sexual promiscuity, of "easiness," of generally not being a "good" woman.[23]

Overall, males tend to shove their mental distress outside of themselves—to "externalize" it, in technical terminology—through "acting out" disorders that use violence, crime, chemicals, or some other generally risky behavior to transform feeling into behavior. Females tend to pull their anguish into themselves—to "internalize" it—in abnormal states of anxiety or mood.[24] Depression, which in its various forms strikes about 10% of women during their lifetimes but fewer than 5% of men, in many ways typifies this pattern of difference. After a first episode of major depression, a disabling, even life-threatening disease, persons of both genders run about the same risk of suffering a second. But, "in study after study, we find that women are two to three times as likely as men" to have that crucial first attack, reports Ellen Frank, Ph.D., professor of psychology and psychiatry at the University of Pittsburgh. This trend is apparent not only in Western countries, but also in 10 nations as diverse as Taiwan and Lebanon, where studies have "found women at least twice as likely to have had one episode of major depression in their lifetime," a ratio that remains remarkably "constant over time."[25]

Opinions vary about what causes these differing rates. Is it some sort of statistical quirk, what statisticians call an "artifact"? Are women more willing to admit that they feel depressed? Could the criteria psychiatrists use to assess depression somehow distort their perceptions? Are there genetic differences? Hormonal differences? Does it have to do with the social statuses women occupy and the social roles they play?

Some recent, important advances in knowledge about depression suggest possibilities. Frank notes one of the most significant: "We now understand that children become depressed," an idea formerly considered "extremely controversial."[26] We also know that the rates of childhood depression show a revealing anomaly: "Prior to age 10," Frank says, "there are virtually no differences between males and females, and in some studies we actually see an excess of depression in boys prior to age 10. But at age 10, rates for girls take off relative to boys, and they never come back again."[27]

For the average girl, that age or the years immediately following represent the gateway to puberty, the time when she exchanges her asexual child's body for the ripening form of a nubile young woman, the era when her emotions must respond for the first time to unknown, and until then unknowable, issues and pressures. Could the onset of the reproductive cycle, with its unaccustomed flood of reproductive hormones, at least partially account for girls' rocketing rates of depression? Numerous authors have suggested links between male-female hormonal differences, which become pronounced at puberty, and various other behavioral differences between the genders. A substantial body of research, for example, links androgens to aggression in a variety of animals, although Donald Pfaff, M.D., professor of neurobiology and behavior at Rockefeller University, notes that "the occasions for the aggression and the target for the aggression might be different between species." Couldn't reproductive hormones influence behaviors as well? Pfaff counsels caution in drawing analogies between humans and other animals; "the linkage of hormone-sensitive forebrain circuits" varies among species "in form and magnitude" and so, therefore, does hormonal impact on behavior. He finds the connection "much less impressive in human beings than it is in many lower mammals." As neurological gender differences get farther from "basic reproductive physiology," they "become smaller and their biological significance is sometimes quite obscure."[28]

Frank is also among those who agree that hormonal changes alone do not suffice to explain gender differences in mental disorders. She suggests another, often overlooked, possibility. A significant prepubertal change, and one long "assumed to be driven by social factors," is that around age 10 or 11 children start staying up later and later. But one study found that "biological factors accounted for all the difference" between older and younger children's bedtimes. Those farther along in puberty, regardless of their chronological age, went to bed the latest. When adult volunteers of both genders, isolated in a bunker from any outside cues as to the time of day, have the chance to schedule their own sleep, women will slumber "on average an hour and a half more for every sleep-wake cycle" that corresponds roughly to a 24-hour day.[29]

Girls, for some as yet unknown reason, thus may well need more sleep than boys. Combining this demand with a later bedtime and the fact that the school day starts at the same early hour regardless of a student's gender could easily produce chronically tired girls "working on an hour and a half sleep deficit" not suffered by boys. "I would argue," Frank concludes, "that this is setting up a kind of fragility in the circadian rhythm" that may partially explain why many more girls than boys of this age become depressed.[30]

But as important a role as physical changes may play during this tumultuous period, girls must deal with powerful social changes as well. "Pubertal and endocrine changes can't be considered in isolation from the social context in which they occur," Frank insists.[31] And one of the starkest social differences dividing the genders is also among the most disturbing. "One of the things we know is that girls are at least twice as vulnerable to childhood sexual abuse as boys," she continues. "In four studies done in quite large samples, we see that rates are almost always at least twice as high for girls as for boys." And other work has decisively established "a direct relationship between childhood sexual abuse and rates of major depression."[32]

But even if the trauma of sexual abuse does not touch a girl, the "social context" of her puberty and adolescence still differs drastically from a boy's. The change from innocent child to attractive sexual object may come quickly, even abruptly, unlike the more gradual changes in physique and social expectations that typically happen to boys. New and troubling uncertainties about her appearance and sexuality increasingly cloud a girl's long-accustomed self-image and social role as she begins to attract an entirely new type of masculine attention. She suffers "a greater discontinuity" than does a boy in "the transition from childhood into adolescence," notes John J. Conger, Ph.D., of the University of Colorado Department of Psychiatry. For boys, their role as maturing adolescents and their road toward manhood, their physical development and their academic and vocational progress, all represent "a continuation or heightening of existing trends." Adolescent girls, however, "are more likely to receive mixed messages than boys, whether about sexuality, appropriate sex roles, or vocational aspirations."[33] So sudden and starkly visible a break with the past puts many girls under tremendous stress. "The young person who . . . finds a reasonable degree of continuity between the competencies, behaviors and values expected of her or him during middle childhood and those expected during puberty and adolescence will also encounter less difficulty in making the adolescent transition," Conger says. "Societies, subcultures and individual families vary widely in this respect."[34]

American society appears rather hard on girls moving into adolescence; the stage constitutes the main exception to the pattern we have observed of greater feminine resilience across the life span. From birth through age 10, boys appear more "vulnerable to both physical and psychosocial stressors" than girls, according to an IOM study of mental disorders.[35] The second decade of life reverses those odds, with girls now showing heightened vulnerability to a host of bodily and psychological ills. By early adulthood, the balance swings back again, with men once more the more vulnerable sex.

ADDICTIONS

A disturbing trend toward increasing—and increasingly early—

use of tobacco, alcohol, and illicit drugs among young women highlights their greater susceptibility to emotional ills during adolescence. Depression or anxiety often afflicts girls who resort to mind-altering substances; whether the contraband chemicals cause the mood disorders or represent a disturbed youngster's attempt at self-medication remains controversial among experts. Male substance abusers much more often suffer antisocial personality disorder than disorders of mood.[36] A girl who responds to the stresses or biochemical changes of adolescence with depression thus runs an increased risk of becoming a substance abuser and even an addict.

Smoking, long a mainly masculine addiction, now poses a particular threat to emotionally vulnerable young women. For many years, and in many countries, a traditional gender gap shaped tobacco use. In Indonesia in 1990, for example, 75% of men smoked, but only 15% of women; in Japan, 70% and 15%, respectively.[37] A similar pattern held in the United States until a generation or so ago. In 1966, for example, only 30% of girls and young women had ever lit up, as compared to 80% of young men. "Before 1960, unquestionably, no matter how you cut the data, more men than women used tobacco products," according to Neil E. Grunberg, Ph.D., professor of psychology at the Uniformed Services University School of Medicine. The pattern held for cigarettes and even more strikingly for cigars, pipes, and chewing tobacco. But then the pattern began to change; by 1980 more women than men were experimenting with tobacco, and by 1990 more teenage girls smoked than boys.[38] Today's smokers, Grunberg observes, are "stereotypically young women, generally middle class to upper middle class, . . . and . . . blue collar men."[39]

Though the great rise in female smoking coincided with epoch-making changes in women's social roles, "it's not just cultural," Grunberg believes. Males and females do not metabolize nicotine identically; evidence suggests that their differing reactions, along with divergent body weight and other factors that affect the molecules' distribution in the body, create different levels of sensitivity in how the two genders react to and metabolize nicotine. Grunberg's own laboratory studied nicotine in rats. "We discovered, to our surprise, that nicotine had a greater effect, dose for dose, in females than in males on body weight and eating behavior, completely consistent with human self reports."[40]

"Everything about the smoking picture is bleak," Henderson laments. "More school girls than school boys are regular smokers by the time they reach tenth grade," and the rise among young women has been particularly sharp.[41] "Cigarette smoking is the habit most likely to drastically change women's overall health status. Unless women stop taking up this habit, lung cancer rates will reach epidemic proportion during the next 20 to 30 years. But lung cancer will be only one of the health consequences."[42] Women smokers can expect to bear more low-birth-weight babies and suffer more heart and lung disease, osteoporosis, and other cancer as well.

Alcohol presents a similarly dismal outlook among young women. More adolescent males than females drink, but the percentage of girls among the very youngest persons drinking to getting drunk—children between 10 and 15—is rising fast.[43] As with cigarettes, this increase portends grim possibilities because alcohol can both devastate a developing fetus and disproportionately injure a female drinker. "We've only recently begun to discover some of the important differences in the impact of drugs and alcohol on males and females," says Frederick K. Goodwin, Ph.D., former administrator of the Alcohol, Drug Abuse and Mental Health Administration. These "important differences" range from the "straightforward"—men's greater ability to metabolize alcohol with stomach enzymes and their resulting lower risk of damage to liver, brain, and other organs—to the "subtle"—interactions with the "highly complex reproductive system in females" as opposed to the "relatively simple reproductive system in males."[44]

Recent research shows that women's stomachs contain less alcohol dehydrogenase, the enzyme that metabolizes alcohol before it enters the bloodstream. For any amount a man and a woman drink, more alcohol reaches her blood. For any amount drunk, she runs a higher risk of alcoholism and liver damage. In women, alcoholism takes a "telescoped course," says Sheila Blume, M.D., medical director of Alcohol, Chemical Dependency, and Compulsive Gambling Programs at South Oaks Hospital, Amityville, New York. "They start later but once they start it moves faster." Females treated for alcoholism also have a higher mortality rate than males.[45]

Whether other drugs of abuse affect the genders differently

remains unclear. "Drug metabolism differences by gender have been poorly studied," found an IOM study on women and health research; from puberty on, though, male metabolic rates outpace those of females.[46] That higher metabolism also helps men lose weight more easily, a physiological fact, the same study found, that combines with our "cultural emphasis on thinness and beauty in women to translate in a higher prevalence of eating disorders, such as anorexia nervosa and bulimia," conditions multiplying in young women but almost nonexistent in men.[47]

BODIES OF EVIDENCE

In her struggle for fashionable emaciation, today's female dieter battles not only an increasingly unrealistic standard of beauty but also the inborn recalcitrance of her own body. "On average, the percent body fat of women is approximately 10 points higher than for men," notes Kirk J. Cureton, Ph.D., professor of exercise science at the University of Georgia and an expert on body composition. Thus the gender obsessed with thinness is also the one that finds it harder to achieve. This difference constitutes more than a cruel genetic joke. Female fat acts decisively in both the economy of reproduction and the physiology of bone. Too little means amenorrhea and premature bone loss.

Besides being fatter than men, women are also less lean. "In adulthood," writes Stanley M. Garn, Ph.D., professor of anthropology and nutrition at the University of Michigan, "the man generally has a larger lean body weight by a ratio of 3:2."[48] This greater muscle mass means that a man is both stronger than a woman of the same size and weight and—to the dismay of female dieters—needs more calories as well.

"At all ages, from the first trimester through the tenth decade," Garn notes, men on average are taller and weigh more than females. "Even during childhood," when boys and girls measure most alike, "the chromosomal XY [or male person] is considerably larger than the chromosomal XX [or female person] of the same physiologic (or skeletal) age."[49] (See Table 2-2.) That's because girls mature sooner than boys and are therefore physiologically "older" at the same chronological age. Men also continue growing into their early twenties, while women stop in their early to mid-teens. Thus, men end up 6 to 7% taller than women

TABLE 2–2 Correspondences Between Male and Female Percentiles for Size and Body Composition in 30- to 39-Year-Old Tecumseh, Michigan, Men and Women

Measure	Male Centiles Corresponding to:	
	Womens' 50th Percentile	Women's 85th Percentile
Stature	2.0	13.1
Weight	7.0	40.6
Fat weight	45.0	88.5
Lean body weight	2.3	18.1
Bone area	3.4	10.4
Cortical area	2.0	14.0
Medullary area	34.4	48.0
Skeletal weight	0.8	8.4

NOTE: This table should be read in the following manner: The 50th percentile for stature in women corresponds to the 2nd percentile in men. The 85th percentile for stature in women corresponds to the 13th percentile for men. Note that the sexes are almost alike in fat weight and skeletal weight.

SOURCE: Institute of Medicine, *Body Composition and Physical Performance: Applications for the Military Services,* 1992, page 211.

"across the socioeconomic range and in different genetic populations," with the additional height concentrated in longer arms and legs—a fact important to designers of driver's seats, machinery, control panels, and the like.[50] Men's skeletons, besides being longer on average, also weigh more by a ratio of 4:3 and contain more calcium than women's.

Women have "smaller skeletons, less bone tissue, smaller bone widths and smaller cortical [core] bone area" than men.[51] One might expect them, Garn suggests, to have more fractures. But until their mid-forties, female skeletons actually prove tougher. The tendency in men toward riskier driving and more dangerous jobs and recreational activities may partially explain this paradox. Both genders lose bone tissue as they age, but for some reason menopause speeds up the process. In her lifetime a woman may lose as much as one-third of the bone she started with in her limb shafts and as much as one-half of her original supply in the shaft ends, the spine, the pelvis, and other flat bones. A man, who had more calcium to begin with, over his lifetime loses one-third less of his larger original endowment.[52] And further worsening older women's chances of avoiding fractures, most women, after a lifetime of exercising less than men, become more sedentary with age and miss out on the weight-bearing exercise known to help preserve bone.[53]

IN CONCLUSION

Like much else about the nature of the genders today, their health differences are, as Churchill said of Russia, "a riddle wrapped in a mystery inside an enigma." Layer upon layer of incomplete insight and spotty data cloud our understanding of how and why women's health experience differs from men's. What's more, we know too little about how the genders' differing endowments set up their characteristic vulnerabilities. Nor have we yet come close to understanding how various treatments and medications differentially affect those distinct physiologies and physiques. And our grasp of the social forces and life experiences at play remains rudimentary. Women's health and the factors that affect it have only begun to attract wide scientific interest. Ten or twenty years hence the writer of a chapter comparable to this one should fill many more pages and need many fewer "not yets" and "unknowns" and "controversials." The true age of discovery has just begun.

NOTES

1. *Disability in America: Toward a National Agenda for Prevention*, 62.
2. IOM 1992 Annual Meeting, 8.
3. Ibid., 8.
4. Ibid., 4.
5. *Women and Health Research: Ethical and Legal Issues of Including Women in Clinical Trials*, Vol. 1, 89.
6. IOM 1992 Annual Meeting, 8-9.
7. Ibid.
8. Ibid., 5.
9. Assessing Future Research Needs: Mental and Addictive Disorders in Women (Transcript), 165.
10. IOM 1992 Annual Meeting, 105.
11. Ibid., 113-4.
12. Ibid., 15.

13. Ibid., 16.
14. *Women and Health Research*, Vol. 1, 89.
15. Ibid.
16. *The Second 50 Years: Promoting Health and Preventing Disability*, 78.
17. IOM 1992 Annual Meeting, 13.
18. *Disability in America*, 67.
19. Ibid., 62.
20. IOM 1992 Annual Meeting, 14-5.
21. *Assessing Future Research Needs: Mental and Addictive Disorders in Women* (Summary), 9.
22. Ibid., 9a.
23. *Broadening the Base of Treatment for Alcohol Problems*, 57.
24. *Reducing Risks for Mental Disorders: Frontiers for Preventive Intervention Research*, 85.
25. IOM 1992 Annual Meeting, 119-20.
26. Ibid., 120-1.
27. Ibid., 121.
28. Ibid., 38.
29. Ibid., 124-5.
30. Ibid.
31. Ibid., 122.
32. Ibid., 126.
33. Assessing Future Research Needs (Transcript), 156.
34. Ibid.
35. *Reducing Risks for Mental Disorders*, 182.
36. Ibid., 8.
37. Assessing Future Research Needs (Transcript), 47.
38. Ibid., 50.
39. Ibid., 49.
40. Ibid., 50.
41. IOM 1992 Annual Meeting, 17-8.
42. Ibid., 17.
43. *Health and Behavior: Frontiers for Research in the Biobehavioral Sciences*, 91.
44. Assessing Future Research Needs (Transcript), 8.
45. Ibid., 219.
46. *Women and Health Research*, Vol. 1, 86.
47. Ibid., 91.
48. *Body Composition and Physical Performance: Applications for the Military Services*, 207.
49. Ibid.
50. Ibid.
51. Ibid., 210.
52. *The Second 50 Years*, 83.
53. *Women and Health Research*, Vol. 1, 90.

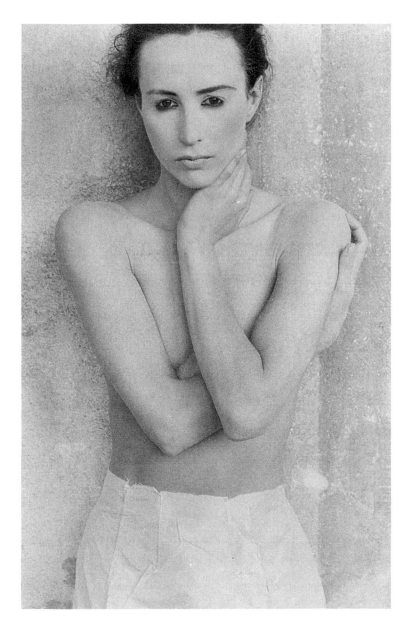

Joyce Tenneson
Kathy (1985)
Silver bromide print
The National Museum of Women in the Arts
Gift of the artist

Roots of Difference

Mapping precisely how and how much women's health differs from men's presents researchers a formidable task. But the challenge of discovering causes for those differences is greater still. Purely physical factors clearly account for some discrepancies; no woman, for example, can develop prostate cancer. Behavior obviously explains others; men have more industrial accidents because more of them work in dangerous industries. But the most intriguing—and probably most revealing—questions fall in between these poles of certainty. Why do women have more osteoporosis but later heart attacks? Why do men suffer more drug addiction but fewer eating disorders?

The origins of various behavioral gender differences—in interests, attainments, social position, and the like—have long sparked debate. For generations, intellectual fashion has swung from nature to nurture and back again. During the decades when the memory remained fresh of World War II atrocities committed in the name of inborn character, scholars and commentators of every kind abjured any explanation that accepted the notion of innate or unchangeable predilections. As those harsh recollections faded, though; as new generations of thinkers began to question their elders' assumptions; and as unprecedented progress in genetics and molecular biology laid bare basic mechanics of human life, the pendulum traveled far back to the nature side. Demonstrated or surmised links between specific genes or chromosomal markers and conditions as diverse as Alzheimer's disease and homosexuality began to dominate discussion. Some enthusiasts now view the imminent mapping of the human genome as a step toward explaining why humans behave as we do.

On the health research front, though, opinion has remained more moderate, moving increasingly toward a consensus that recognizes both biology and behavior. Advances in genetics have, of course, strongly influenced recent thinking about the origins of disorders from breast and colon cancer to schizophrenia. But in a seeming paradox, many such purported biological connections seem also to suggest important roles for environment and behavior. Heredity appears to set up a variety of specific susceptibilities. Circumstance then may or may not transform them into full-blown disorders.

Gender differences in physical and mental well-being, according to this view, thus mirror the complex interplay of bodily endowment and life experience. Males' and females' distinctive physiological properties can each produce characteristic vulnerabilities. Their divergent life courses exert differing stressors. Together, nature and nurture mold an individual's—and a gender's—total health profile. Neither factor alone offers a complete explanation. Together, though, they provide useful insights into the dynamics of health and illness.

Indeed, researchers have only recently begun to appreciate the true subtlety and multiplicity of the connections between body and behavior, between genetics, physiology, and personal history. Some ties are as simple and straightforward as men's higher incidence of lung cancer, which obviously reflects their historically greater consumption of cigarettes. Other connections are as complicated as the influence of gonadal hormones on various functions not directly involved in reproduction. The way an individual handles stress, for example, influences such important aspects of health as immunity and blood pressure. Recent studies of the hormonal system controlling the stress response, for example, reveal close links to the system that regulates the reproductive hormones.

Thus "the consequences of stress appear to differ in males and females," states Bruce McEwen, professor of endocrinology at Rockefeller University, noting a potentially very significant, but as yet incompletely understood, gender divergence. Primate studies even suggest that "the female brain may actually be protected from some destructive effects of stress," he adds, "perhaps through mechanisms involving gonadal hormones, perhaps through other mechanisms." He submits that "wear and tear of stress hormones and sex hormones . . . can actually wear out structures and systems in the brain. . . . Since brain cells are not regenerated during adult life, this can lead to the actual wearing of brain structures and contribute to the rate of the aging process."[1] Huda Akil, Ph.D., of the Mental Health Research Institute at the University of Michigan, whose research has explored the ties between females' reproductive and stress hormone responses, notes that scientists' assumption that these systems are separate has helped obscure the link.[2] Adds Maureen Henderson, "the interplay of reproductive and other hormones has to be a central theme and top priority for allocation of research resources."[3]

Another connection deserving further investigation, experts agree, links gender differences in brain structure or function with vulnerability to a variety of psychological and cognitive conditions. Mental and addictive disorders were formerly thought to arise mainly from emotional causes. But increasingly strong evidence now suggests that physiology plays an influential role in the genders' differing patterns. "The more we study gender differences, the more we find physiologically significant differences in brain structure, in brain chemistry, and in peripheral areas such as liver metabolism of hormones and drugs," states McEwen.[4]

Some of these distinctions focus on the way the brain is organized, some on the mechanisms that activate its various structures. Disparities such as boys' higher rates of learning disabilities, for example, persuade McEwen that "there's a fundamental difference in cerebral development that can lead or predispose more males" to show such problems. Various other features, including "differences at the level of autonomic and more vegetative and regulatory functions" and the effects of hormones on various neurological systems, are known to affect the actions of certain psychoactive drugs.[5]

These discrepancies lead McEwen to the conclusion that "in all studies of drug effects, addictive disorders, mental disorders . . . males and females, men and women, are in fact two distinctly different populations and should be treated as such . . . until evidence shows that it's not necessary to further consider gender differences." Still, he adds, "we know very little up to this point about the underlying mechanisms. . . . There's a great need for further investigation."[6]

Just how great is that need becomes obvious when we consider the tremendous power of those "underlying mechanisms." "Complex differences between the two sexes ultimately stem from very minor or simple differences" during embryonic development, says Jean Wilson, M.D., professor of medical sciences at the University of Texas Southwest Medical Center and a leader in hormone research. Scientists know a great deal about the biology of this process, but "in some ways we know nothing. The challenge for the 90s is understanding the behavioral and functional consequences of these small differences during embryogenesis, and how these differences are amplified by sociological, psychological, and secondary endocrine effects." The task of tracking gender differences to their origins "is going to be more complicated than what we've accomplished to date."[7]

CULTURAL CONSIDERATIONS

Clearly, physiology alone cannot answer questions like why males and females suffer such different patterns of mental illness, any more than it totally accounts for variations in physical ones. "I would underscore the need to integrate the biological and psychosexual studies," says Ellen Frank, Ph.D., professor of psychiatry at the University of Pittsburgh. "All of these disorders and problems are happening within one skin, and unless we study the same individual from both perspectives, we will never understand how the vulnerability factors fit together with the stressors. It's almost . . . pointless to look only at one dimension or the other. Until we fit these pieces together, we will never understand what is happening."[8]

Behavioral, social, and psychological differences between the genders thus require analysis as painstaking as any in the biological realm. Within many societies, as we have repeatedly noted, female health differs from male. But between societies, women's or men's physical or mental well-being can also vary sharply, revealing the extreme importance of specific social and economic conditions. In developed nations like the United States, researchers ponder the mystery of why women live so much longer than men, weighing possibilities ranging from immunity to employment.

In many other countries, though, investigators confront a quite different mystery, the one that Susan Scrimshaw, Ph.D., of the UCLA School of Public Health, terms the whereabouts of the "missing women, . . . the issue of skewed sex ratios in countries where women receive less than equal treatment." European and North American censuses find 96 males for every 100 females, with the gap widening as people age. But in the developing world, this ratio "flips," in Scrimshaw's word. India counts 93.5 females to every 100 males; Bangladesh, 94 females to every 100 males; and Egypt, 105 males to every 100 females.[9] By U.S. standards, therefore, "over 1 million Egyptian women are missing, victims of higher than biologically expected mortality throughout the life span."[10]

In addition to the Egyptian women prematurely dead—at least by North American standards—large numbers of their living female fellow citizens suffer disabilities that relate to pregnancy but are relatively rare in the United States. For every Egyptian woman who dies in pregnancy or childbirth, an estimated 10 to 15 others "survive severe, life-threatening morbidity," Scrimshaw states. A study in one Egyptian city found more than half the women suffering reproductive tract infections, with equally large numbers living with anemia and uterine prolapse. "We don't have studies of this depth in other countries, but we do have the same kinds of figures for missing women," Scrimshaw observes. "The life expectancy of women in the northern countries, . . . Europe and the U.S., is 30 years longer than for women in developing countries."[11]

The apparently "natural" longevity advantage of American women thus emerges as at least a partial product of their widespread access to adequate nutrition and safe maternity and gynecological care. Throughout the developing world, surveys show, more than half of women want no more children or want them more widely spaced than is possible without effective contraception or access to safe abortion. Many women die from botched illegal abortions, from births separated by less than a year, or from childbearing either very early or very late in one's life. Half of Egypt's annual mortality, for example, consists of women older than 30 attempting to bear child number three, four, five, or even higher.[12] Other American gender differences that appear equally "natural" to us—perhaps our discrepant rates of heart disease or cancer, for example—may well also arise from social rather than medical disparities likewise obscured by a particular culture's notion of what constitutes the "normal."

Many such disparities clearly exist. "We know of no culture that has said articulately that there is no difference between men and women except in the way they contribute to the next generation; that otherwise, in all respects, they are simply human beings with varying gifts," said the anthropologist Margaret Mead.[13] For Scrimshaw, this statement by her scholarly mentor emphasizes the "one underlying cultural theme [that] emerged with surprising consistency and intensity" from the scientific literature on women's health worldwide: "the inequalities."[14] In nearly every culture known, she notes, the genders have unequal access to social and economic resources; unequal family responsibilities and work roles; unequal abilities to control expenditures, fertility, and time; unequal power to exercise their own choices.

Nor, in evaluating how life experience affects health, can we regard any given society's female populations as uniform. Who represents the "typical" American woman facing "normal" health threats? A farm wife exposed to pesticides and fertilizers and stranded scores of miles from the closest primary care? An inner-city welfare mother in danger of HIV infection from a drug-using partner and dependent on Medicaid and a nearby emergency room for what care she manages to get? A thirty-something single attorney subject to intense job stress and downtown air pollution? A college student experimenting with recreational drugs and casual sex? A prosperous suburban housewife? A single mother employed as a factory hand? A poor immigrant from a developing nation who resorts first to a practitioner of her homeland's folk medicine? A nursing home resident? Even in countries far less diverse than our own, even in societies where tradition still provides the script for most biographies, "women" do not constitute a unitary mass. Ethnic affiliation, social class, and economic position everywhere mold personal experience.

Age also plays a crucial role in health status, its influence varying according to an individual's particular social setting and life history. "If women have differential access to food, work and health care," Scrimshaw notes, "it is more different at some stages of their lives than others. . . . Women's roles are not static but dynamic."[15] In some places a pregnant woman must eschew various foods; in others she is stuffed with special delicacies. In some places a young girl risks her life by smiling at a man outside her family, but a postmenopausal grandmother moves freely about the town. In some places, women are pressed to bear children in their mid-teens and become matriarchs by their forties. In others, women devote their first three decades to education and career and only commence motherhood in their mid-thirties.

The cultural norms of many countries expose females in other parts of the world to health risks quite different from those faced by females in North America. Where poor parents value male offspring markedly more than female, fewer girl babies survive infancy. Where respectability requires female circumcision, girls suffer bleeding and infection both at the childhood ceremony and repeatedly later on during sexual intercourse and childbirth. Where men and boys have first crack at the most nutritious foods, growing girls and pregnant or nursing women may lack needed nourishment. Where standards of modesty restrict the movements of postpubescent girls and young wives, earning money or obtaining health care may present serious obstacles. Where women lack birth control, many closely spaced pregnancies fill the years between late adolescence and middle age. Where pregnancies are frequent and nutrition inadequate, anemia weakens mothers and complicates deliveries. Where medical attention is scarce, many expectant mothers join the half-million worldwide who die each year from problems related to pregnancy.[16] Where wives bear heavier responsibilities than their husbands for cooking, cleaning, marketing, child care, tending kitchen gardens and small animals, and working in the fields, they suffer increased fatigue. Where forming dung into fuel cakes or washing and cooking in contaminated water are normal housewifely tasks, parasites are normal housewifely ailments. Where married men customarily visit prostitutes, their wives routinely contract venereal diseases. Where widows have no support but their children, the childless live in penury.

To understand any gender variation in health patterns that we observe, therefore, Scrimshaw insists we must first ask a basic question: "Why women?" What is there about their lives that opens them to a specific possibility? What particular realities of their time and place produce a certain combination of vulnerability and stressor? The answer may come from any realm that touches women's lives, from biochemistry to fashion.

In the spring and summer of 1980, for example, exactly that combination of factors challenged American public health officials. Hundreds of women, mostly previously healthy whites between 15 and 19, came down with a sudden, sometimes deadly, but theretofore rare illness that only two years earlier had been named toxic shock syndrome (TSS). The patient's temperature shot up, her heart raced, her blood pressure dropped, her breathing became rapid, and she broke out in a rash. The skin peeled from her palms and soles. She became lethargic. Sometimes her kidneys began to fail. In several dozen cases, the patient died.

By September of that year, investigators had found a strong association between TSS, the bacterium *Staphylococcus aureus* (an organism already well-known as the culprit in a number of human diseases), and the use of tampons during menstruation, especially a superabsorbent brand known as Rely. The scientific evidence then available did not permit an IOM committee studying the outbreak to identify either the exact mechanism connecting these sanitary products to the disease or the reasons that the condition preferentially targeted young whites. It did conclude, however, that "a marked reduction in the number of cases would be expected in the absence of tampon use."[17]

Put in other words, this finding meant that the dictates of fashion, combined with advances in fiber technology, had placed American women at risk for a potentially deadly disease. In 1980, U.S. tampon sales topped 5 billion, with 70% of the nation's 50 million menstruating women choosing internal protection. Most teenagers used napkins for their initial menstrual periods but switched to tampons within two years.[18]

Disposable sanitary napkins first appeared on the American market after World War I, when firms making surgical dressings sought replacements for their vanished military customers. Until then, women had contented themselves with diapers or squares of cloth, confident that bustles and petticoats hid any telltale outlines. The more form-fitting fashions of the late 1920s and early 1930s created demand for protection that did not show, and manufacturers responded with devices that could be worn internally. Similar esthetic constraints had led women in ancient Greece and Rome to insert cylinders of rolled wool into their vaginas.

Cotton tampons hit the American market in the early 1930s. By the late 1970s, newly developed superabsorbent synthetic fibers promised to make them ever more reliable and long-wearing. For reasons not fully understood, though, these new, improved models also increased certain women's vulnerability to severe staph infections.[19] Experts do not know whether the racial and age differentials observed in TSS cases relate to differing patterns of sanitary protection or to some other factor.[20] Clearly, though, solving this puzzle would require a very detailed knowledge of women's daily habits. The collection of this kind of information has hardly begun.

MAPPING LIVES

Gender differences that affect health start out small and begin to expand in early childhood. By adolescence, American boys and girls are well along the diverging paths that will carry them to their very different adulthoods as men and women. Puberty is one of the major milestones along the route, the first of several major life transitions that demarcate American lives. Like the passages to parenthood, the post-reproductive years, and old age, adolescence involves its own distinct health risks. How an individual responds to them helps establish physical, psychological, and behavioral patterns that can significantly affect later health.

Each new life stage also imposes particular developmental demands, as an individual adjusts to new roles, responsibilities, opportunities, and limits. Meeting these in a health-enhancing way is an important challenge of development, one complicated or eased by the individual's circumstances and the expectations of those around her. The task is often difficult. "Most of us were brought up on a naive psychoanalytic notion of development as a kind of continuous linear model," says Dr. Bertram Cohler, professor of psychology at the University of Chicago. "In fact, development is more like a series of wrenching transformations across the course of life" [21]

That course begins in childhood, a period when boys and girls traditionally faced quite similar health issues. "In earlier times, the childhood diseases that people studied had very little to do with gender," notes Eleanor Maccoby, Ph.D., professor emeritus of psychology at Stanford

University and a leading researcher in the development of gender differences. In the days before vaccinations and antibiotics had wiped out measles, mumps, whooping cough, rheumatic fever, polio, and the many other contagions that afflicted children, "the disease entities, their diagnosis and treatment were generally the same for the two sexes."[22]

But what used to be called "childhood illnesses" have all but vanished from American childhoods. A new set of ailments now poses the major threat to our young. Violence, depression, drug abuse, eating disorders and the like differ from old-time maladies in three ways: they strike in adolescence, they preferentially target one gender or the other, and they have, in Maccoby's words, "a more behavioral component," resulting, at least in part, from the choices that youngsters make, often under the influence of peers.[23] Researchers have yet to pin down the origin of these problems. Clearly, though, boys' and girls' quite different experiences in and after puberty contribute significantly.

But do the divergent patterns that produce the first significant gender-based health distinctions actually arise in adolescence? Or does their source, as Maccoby's research suggests, lie much earlier in the life span? "I want to argue," she asserts, "that the behavior patterns that so importantly affect adolescent health have their roots in childhood, and that the relevant developmental history differs for boys and girls."[24] As far back as the preschool years, she believes, males and females inhabit gradually diverging subcultures. The attitudes and behaviors they learn help set up the quite disparate vulnerabilities that emerge a decade or more later.

ROLES AND RITUALS

This process of gender differentiation begins very subtly. Until the age of 2 or so, boys and girls are "remarkably alike," differing by personal temperament much more than by gender-related traits.[25] By age 3, however, children know which gender they belong to and have begun the long process of figuring out what that membership means. From about age 4, given the opportunity, they begin favoring playmates of their own gender.

Distinctive styles of interaction now begin to emerge within the all-male and all-female groups. Research among primates has shown a similar pattern of segregated play groups, with juvenile males doing lots of roughhousing and juvenile females mostly stepping aside to avoid the ruckus. This suggests to Maccoby that "something biological" may lie behind the desire for separation. But the habit of clustering by gender, whatever its basis, "then takes on a life of its own, that is stamped by the culture" in which the children live.[26] A small biological divergence, perhaps in energy level or aggressiveness, and possibly based on boys' higher androgen levels, thus becomes magnified by customs and values into increasingly significant behavioral differences.[27]

In the culture of the American schoolyard and playing field, "boys are more concerned with dominance issues, with who is tougher," developing "dominance hierarchies that are quite stable." Girls' cliques, meanwhile, are "less hierarchical and their play more integrated by a joint script," Maccoby says. They "increasingly use polite suggestions and questions such as 'Why don't we . . .?' or 'Wouldn't you like to . . .?' to influence their playmates." Boys use more and more "direct commands, such as 'Bring me that.' "[28] With their tough-guy style and their focus on heroics (both their own and those of sports stars or superheroes), boys become increasingly impervious to the gentler style of persuasion that works in the more harmonious female play groups.

By grade school, the habit of sorting themselves by gender has come to dominate children's social life. Male play emphasizes dominance and competition. Boys often gather in large groups for organized games that use well-defined rules to determine winners and losers. They brag, heckle, joke, bluff, misbehave to demonstrate their daring, show off for one another, and generally try to appear at least as rugged as the next guy. Girls, meanwhile, gather in sets of twos or threes, where they endeavor to create closeness. "Speech serves a more egoistic function among boys and a more socially binding one among girls," Maccoby notes.[29] As puberty approaches, girls begin to spend more and more time speculating about romance. Boys, meanwhile, expand their repertoire of tough talk to the subject of sex, recounting purported exploits, sharing pornography, and telling dirty jokes.

Contact with the opposite sex once again becomes socially legitimate, although most youngsters still spend their time overwhelmingly with friends of their own gender. Among themselves, boys and girls continue getting along in their accustomed ways. "Girl-girl friendships are typically more intimate, mutually supportive," Maccoby observes. "When they talk to each other, their style is more sociable, less confrontational. Males continue to play to their male audiences with risk-taking displays."[30]

PROBLEMS AT PUBERTY AND BEYOND

There is now, however, something decidedly new under the youngsters' suns: contacts with the opposite sex that carry potentially significant health consequences. "When young boys and girls emerge from the gender-segregated social groupings of childhood and begin to interact with each other, the two sexes are not on a level playing field," Maccoby says. Entering the age of budding sexuality, girls come equipped with the cooperative habits of their social set, and a mode of persuasion that sounds tentative and unconvincing to boys accustomed to a more aggressive, combative style. And "of course," Maccoby notes, "the implications for being sexually active are different for the two sexes."[31]

Who can get pregnant is only one of the many important differences. Another is the "asymmetry in the importance of physical appearance."[32] Though nearly all youngsters hope the opposite sex finds them attractive, boys give looks more weight in choosing a partner than do girls. Squiring a beauty adds a great deal to a boy's social stature. For girls, the mere fact of having a boyfriend may well outweigh the details of his appearance. Her wardrobe, her figure, her hair, and her skin become major female preoccupations. "These concerns are so central for young girls that they often take priority over other girls, and even academically gifted girls can lose self-esteem, lose interest in their school work, and become depressed if they think they are too fat or otherwise unattractive," Maccoby says.[33]

Not only a girl's grades but also her health can suffer permanent damage from the relentless demands of appearance. The ideal of the muscular, athletic man may be "difficult enough for boys to reach," Conger says, but today's archetype of slender feminine beauty is "an impossible one for girls." Growing into their adult bodies, boys put on weight mainly as lean muscle tissue, but girls gain mostly fat. "Thus, whereas physical maturation brings boys closer to the masculine ideal, for most girls it means the development away from what is currently considered beautiful," Conger laments. "Not surprisingly, then, girls are far more likely than boys to be dissatisfied with their appearance and body image, particularly in the early adolescent years."[34]

Fighting their natural bent in search of an unattainable silhouette sets up girls, especially those developing earlier than their friends or "genetically programmed to be heavier than the svelte ideal," for eating disorders.[35] The right combination of biology and psychology can turn a teenager's normal concern about her figure into anorexia nervosa or bulimia. Nearly all young women diet at some time or other, but only a minority of the biologically vulnerable appear to tip over into these life-threatening exaggerations of weight control, says Dr. Katherine Halmi, professor of psychiatry at Cornell University. When a susceptible person begins dieting, "various other physiological effects cascade" toward a full-fledged illness. "Disturbed perceptions of hunger and satiety" distort eating patterns. As the pounds fall away from an increasingly emaciated body, victims develop a satisfying feeling of control, although, "in reality, they have lost all control. Even if they want to, they cannot start eating normally."[36]

"Three major neurotransmitters, serotonin, norepinephine and dopamine, are heavily involved in the hypothalamus in regulating eating behavior," Halmi explains. "There is accumulating evidence that bulimia patients have a disregulation of serotonin function," and "that bulimics have a disregulation of norepinephrine"—imbalances that also affect hormone responses "in producing the full-blown syndrome."[37] Depression and irritability set in as starvation advances. Anxiety, personality disorders, and other psychiatric ailments plague many of these young women as well.

Culture's contribution consists of some impossible contradictions. Women between 18 and 40 on average weigh more than they did three decades ago, a fact that in itself encourages dieting. At the same time, the media's standard of fashionable weight has fallen sharply. And advertisements for sweet, fatty foods barrage today's teens. Families can also unwittingly foster troubled eating. A genetic element is likely, given the higher incidence of the disorders among the relatives of bulimics and anorexics; these disorders, Halmi says, "breed true."[38] But Conger also notes psychological factors. "In addition to being overly involved emotionally, overprotective and rigid," parents "appear to be unduly conscious of appearance and to attach special meaning to food and eating. The first generation of daughters of the first group of women who went to Weight Watchers had an unusually high incidence of bulimia. I don't know if that's an advertisement or not."[39]

Either way, other advertisements seem to help insecure girls worried about their weight adopt another health-destroying habit, smoking. Teens of both genders experiment with cigarettes, but by tenth grade more girls than boys regularly light up. Many girls believe that smoking helps control weight. Scientific evidence also indicates that "smoking is a momentary reliever of anxiety and stress," Maccoby says.[40] Athletics may encourage boys to eschew tobacco after their initial attempts. But if present trends persist, soon the United States could have, for the first time in its history, more females smoking than males.[41]

But just as a remorseless teen culture may push girls toward behaviors indicating mental illness, it may guide boys into actions that mask similar problems. Delinquency and drunkenness, some experts believe, may be mood disorders in macho disguise; although they may well express similar feelings of worthlessness and hopelessness, they are not currently classified as symptoms of depression. Among Amish adolescents, says Paula J. Clayton, M.D., of the Department of Psychiatry at University Hospital in Minneapolis, such outlets do not exist; "alcoholism and drugs are culturally prohibited and acts of violence and crime are infrequent." The sect's boys and girls suffer mood disorders at similar rates. Adding together the delinquency and depression rates for America's mainstream adolescents also produces similar incidence levels for both genders.[42]

With the passage to adulthood, though, as the demanding male role begins to close in on young men, the tables may turn. Social expectations may now cause more males to appear among the ranks of the mentally ill. Schizophrenia, for example, often strikes in early adulthood and frequently takes a less favorable course in men than women. Male schizophrenics spend more time in hospitals, are readmitted more often, and generally do worse in their work and social lives. Might not one reason be that families feel differently toward schizophrenic sons and daughters and those feelings affect treatment decisions? Although the disease's severity may actually differ in males and females, Jill Goldstein, assistant professor of psychiatry at Harvard University Medical School, believes that "social role expectations" might also contribute.[43]

The strictures of adult roles take their toll on feminine health, as well. "The impact of sexuality and the concept of childbearing" are "strongly different" for the two genders, Maccoby observes.[44] The overriding disparity is society's assumption that the mother will bear the major burden of rearing the children, a responsibility that often translates into lesser career prospects, financial and psychological dependence on a mate, and willingness to subordinate one's own interests to others'.

The female role has also traditionally dictated that girls and women take less part in sports than boys and men. And even for those active in youth, physical activity tends to decline as one advances into womanhood. "From 45 onwards, when fitness really begins to count, less than one third of women exercise regularly and less than one in ten exercises intensively and regularly," Henderson notes. Rates of exercise "go downhill instead of uphill as women get older." Bone mass, cardiovascular fitness, stamina, and mental attitude all suffer as a consequence. Do women's "four bad years" at the end of life result as much from "earlier social conditioning as [from] ill health"?[45]

IN CONCLUSION

Such a question appears at once obvious and unanswerable. Clearly, choices made throughout the life span affect health at every age. Just as clearly, we do not now know, and perhaps never will, just how much one's physical and mental state depends on culture and experience and how much on physiological and anatomical traits, both those unique to the individual and those shared with an entire gender. Armed with our ever-advancing biological knowledge and a powerful new life-span perspective, investigators are just beginning to ask the right questions. Answers lie far in the future.

NOTES

1. Assessing Future Research Needs: Mental and Addictive Disorders in Women (Transcript), 261.

2. Ibid., 121.
3. IOM 1992 Annual Meeting, 19.
4. Assessing Future Research Needs (Transcript), 260.
5. Ibid.
6. Ibid.
7. IOM 1992 Annual Meeting, 36.
8. Assessing Future Research Needs (Transcript), 288.
9. Scrimshaw (1991), 4.
10. Ibid., 5.
11. Ibid.
12. *Science and Babies: Private Decisions, Public Dilemmas*, 54-5.
13. Quoted in Scrimshaw (1991), 2.
14. Ibid.
15. Ibid., 6.
16. Ibid., 12.
17. *Toxic Shock Syndrome: An Assessment of Current Information and Future Research Needs*, 85.
18. Ibid., 47-8.
19. Ibid., 45-7.
20. Ibid., 56.
21. Assessing Future Research Needs (Transcript), 166.
22. IOM 1992 Annual Meeting, 73.
23. Ibid.
24. Ibid.
25. Ibid.
26. Ibid., 94-5.
27. Ibid., 95.
28. Ibid., 77.
29. Ibid., 80.
30. Ibid., 82.
31. Ibid., 74.
32. Ibid., 83.
33. Ibid., 84.
34. Assessing Future Research Needs (Transcript), 157.
35. Ibid., 158.
36. Ibid., 212.
37. Ibid., 214-5.
38. Ibid., 210-1.
39. Ibid., 158.
40. IOM 1992 Annual Meeting, 90.
41. Ibid., 55.
42. Ibid., 187.
43. Assessing Future Research Needs (Transcript), 202.
44. Ibid., part 2, 46.
45. IOM 1992 Annual Meeting, 14.

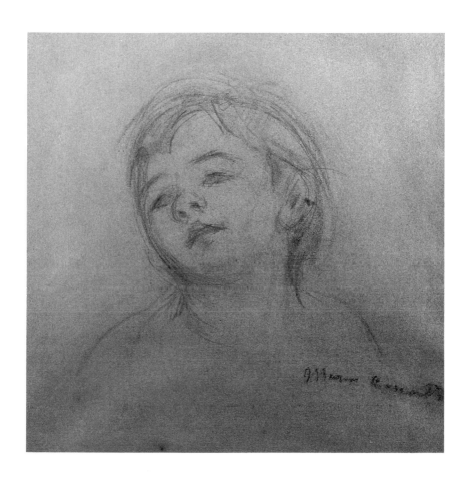

Mary Cassatt
Sketch of Denise's Daughter (ca. 1905)
Charcoal on paper
The National Museum of Women in the Arts
Gift of Mrs. Kitty Taquey in memory of her father, Mr. Albert McVitty

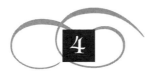

Health Through the
Life Span:
The First Two Decades

C arved into the granite lintel over the entrance to the National Archives in Washington, D.C., is a line from Shakespeare's *The Tempest*: "What's past is prologue." The Bard intended the phrase to illuminate human nature; the builders of the nation's document repository, to affirm the importance of historical study. But the motto just as aptly encapsulates a central fact about physical and mental health: today's condition derives from yesterday's and affects tomorrow's.

To an enormous extent, perhaps even greater than among men, the motto holds true for women. A woman's personal history—her weight at birth, the timing of major life events, various choices she makes, the pressures that impinge on her—casts a long shadow over her physical and mental well-being throughout her lifetime. Did she develop a taste for athletics in childhood? Did her menarche come early or late? Did she succumb to peer culture during adolescence? Has she had few or many sexual partners? Has she used safe and effective contraceptives? Did she build strong bones during youth? Did she bear children as a young woman, in middle age, or not at all? Did she receive hormone treatment at meno-

---

The discussion of the life-span perspective as it applies to women's health derives from the IOM report *In Her Lifetime: Female Morbidity and Mortality in Sub-Saharan Africa*.

pause? Does she survive her husband? Each of these facts, though seemingly minor in itself, nonetheless can influence such large matters as how long she lives, how well she feels at various points in her life, and what ailments befall her.

As biographers and novelists have long known, the perspective of a person's entire life span affords a special insight into the ages and stages that compose his or her allotment of individual days. Medical researchers, however, have only lately come around to this insight and have only in recent years begun to appreciate fully the power of the long view to clarify health conditions, particularly of women.

Until not very long ago, for example, the idea of pregnancy used to distort analyses of women's health even more than the fact of it alters their silhouettes. The capacity to conceive, carry, birth, and nurse healthy babies, or to efficiently avoid doing so, focused interest—as an expectant mother's belly draws attention from her arms, legs, even her face—on a single, transitory aspect of her being, to the near exclusion of many more enduring features.

Unlike the older, pregnancy-centered view, the newer life span perspective regards a woman's experience as happening first and foremost to *her*, not to or because of or for the benefit of anyone else. Her body, her health, in this view, are first and foremost hers, and only secondarily the fetal environment of her offspring. We can easily recognize this person-centered perspective, of course, from the study of the health of men. Historically, very few researchers have considered the male body primarily as a mechanism for producing healthy sperm or providing support for growing children, even though numerous experiences and influences can affect the ability to create or ejaculate viable sperm cells and perform parental duties. Nor have scientists usually evaluated the events that befall a man mainly in relation to their effect on those capacities. Affording him a long and satisfying life has always seemed a sufficient end in itself.

In this same spirit, we approach the female life span, especially as lived in the United States in the last years of the twentieth century. In a nation as large and varied as our own, as we've seen, and among a gender undergoing such rapid and far-reaching social change, there can be no "typical" American life. But because, as we noted in Chapter 1, health is the intersection of each person's innate endowment and his or her life experience, and because all women share important inborn features, we can expect to find certain characteristic patterns among the vast array of individual experiences. By its nature the female body passes through certain distinctive—and distinctively sensitive—periods, wherever a woman happens to live. Onto this genetic template, American culture also imposes its own particular pressures.

A second concept, the sensitive period, will also help us illuminate the connections in female lives. Every organism goes through a number of such times, during which, because of physical, emotional, developmental, or other factors, it is "especially vulnerable to an event such as sensory deprivation, malnutrition, or exposure to toxins," according to an IOM report on child development. To focus on a simple and especially fleeting example, intrauterine infections generally have their severest effects during the fetus's first three months of development; an identical disease striking later in the pregnancy does much less damage.

Other such crucial points occur at various stages of the life span. Discovering when, and which, events trigger harmful consequences, and what factors affect the organism's susceptibility or resistance, and how adverse effects can be overcome today constitutes "one of the key issues for clinicians and researchers," the IOM report notes.[1] Because the sensitive period concept arose first in animal studies, it "has traditionally been associated with the prenatal period and infancy"; experience has proven it "applicable to all stages of development," however.[2] As we journey through American women's lives, we will see this concept's explanatory power again and again.

THE EARLY YEARS

For the better part of this century, the great majority of all American lives have begun in hospitals, where the technical ability to cope with complicated births has reached unparalleled heights. Even very small or sick infants now have an excellent chance of surviving birth and the period immediately following. In fact, unless born to a mother who fails to receive adequate prenatal care or who abuses substances, American babies face relatively few dangers, especially as compared to children in developing countries. If she grows up in a family that enjoys emotional stability, an adequate income, and appropriate medical attention, further-more, a healthy young American girl normally avoids serious medical problems and deprivations. In recent years, though, this all-important "if" has become increasingly problematic for far too many youngsters. Not only do today's children include an unprecedented number living in single-parent homes, they also have, for the first time in American history, the highest poverty rate of any age group.[3]

Thanks to vaccinations and antibiotics, children who get ad-equate medical attention also escape the many contagions that within living memory were common enough to merit the term "childhood dis-eases." Polio no longer terrorizes swimming pools and summer camps. Measles, mumps, whooping cough, and scarlet fever no longer race through schoolrooms. Rheumatic heart disease no longer condemns kids to months in bed. Ear infections no longer destroy their hearing.

But even as infectious disease has been largely conquered, sig-nificant—and possibly growing—numbers of children still succumb to mental, emotional, and behavioral disorders, including some, like learning disabilities and attention deficits, only relatively recently identified and understood. During the preschool and elementary years, these afflictions strike fewer girls than boys, although girls at every age face a higher risk of sexual abuse—at least twice as high, according to studies.[4] As if to illus-trate the sensitive period concept, in fact, childhood referrals for psychia-tric and psychological help peak at certain ages—around 4 and then again between 7 and 9. Such times each mark a "transitional stage" in the child's growth, when "accelerations in physical or cognitive development or rapid changes in parental expectation and general societal demands . . . require new adjustments," Conger observes.[5]

And so, with the major physical threats essentially solved for American youngsters covered by decent health insurance, the big health considerations in the early years now involve more developmental is-sues—laying the groundwork, both physical and emotional, for long-term well-being. Habits developed in childhood—eating a healthful diet, for example, or practicing good oral hygiene, or getting lots of exercise—can bring lifelong benefits. Equally important are the self-image and interper-sonal skills that children acquire. As we have already noted, boys and girls begin segregating themselves as toddlers. By first grade, Maccoby found, they are choosing playmates from their own gender 11 times as often as from the opposite one.[6]

These play groups develop styles that can crucially affect health when kids enter adolescence. Maccoby notes that girls learn to be "reciprocal and responsive with boys. . . . They listen to what a boy says and answer him and maybe do what be wants and expect him to do what they want." But boys listen to each other and "are seldom influenced by the response that they get from a girl." For their part, "girls don't like to play with someone they can't reciprocate with." They "back off from play with boys."[7]

This "backing off" tends to remove girls from the games and playing fields stereotyped as male. "The girls get the territories that are left over from what the boys have grabbed," Maccoby goes on. "The boys get the big areas for their ball games, and the girls are on the edges," jumping rope or skipping across hopscotch boards, or bouncing their small pink balls to counting rhymes.[8] Hours and years at the line of scrimmage or in the batter's box or under the hoop teach boys the skills and satisfactions of strenuous physical activity. Many girls, meanwhile, still pass through childhood convinced that exercise is something that other people do. For the rest of their lives, they are more sedentary than males.

Even more important than what their play teaches about exercise, though, is what each gender learns about the other and about relationships in general. Girls become expert at building friendships around talk, persuasion, and sharing both confidences and leadership. Boys build theirs around shared activities, kidding, and friendly competition for dominance. Boys spend much less time talking and almost none sharing confidences. Thus, as girls enter a period when their present and future health crucially depends on the influence of males, they come at a very considerable disadvantage.

ADOLESCENCE

The passage from childhood to adolescence is among the most complex and variable that Americans make. In the first place, it happens at very different times for different individuals. "Normal" children of the same age can enter puberty as much as two or three years apart. From the fifth to the ninth grade, any given class includes youngsters at vastly different points in the transition. In general, girls who develop on the early side experience more stress than their later-blooming classmates.

Also crucial to the experience, Conger believes, is a highly variable factor: "how nearly optimal the young person's development has been during earlier age periods." A child who had "trusting, secure relationships with caretakers during infancy and early childhood and who is able to achieve competency in physical, cognitive and social skills and a positive sense of self during middle childhood, will be better prepared to weather the demands of puberty and adolescence than one who has not." But these days, alas, a decent childhood is far from a foregone conclusion. "One of the tragedies of our time," Conger goes on, "is the mounting number of children who have been denied both of these essential psychological building blocks, and who in all too many instances have also been denied basic health and neurobiological integrity, whether as a result of maternal drug use, malnutrition, exposure to toxic environmental agents or physical abuse and neglect."[9]

But ready or not, girls must face puberty whenever it happens, ushering many of them into a period of turmoil and complex new vulnerabilities. Their bodies change from children's to women's; their images of themselves, and others' images of them, change just as drastically, permanently, and fundamentally. They become—at first physically, and then, with varying degrees of difficulty, emotionally as well—overtly sexual beings. More specifically, in the context of modern American adolescence, they become sex objects and sexual actors. Boys are also making a similar shift, if a year or two later. But the impact appears more negative for girls than for boys. Girls of this age "begin to develop an awareness of their inferior social status," both sexually and generally, Frank observes.[10]

What's more, there is a "profound asymmetry in sexuality itself," Maccoby notes—an imbalance that goes far beyond the obvious fact that only females get pregnant.[11] Adolescent girls find themselves disadvantaged in a number of other ways. They are physically smaller than boys and headed for a less prestigious adult role. They suffer rape—and the constraints on mobility imposed by the fear of rape—to a far greater extent than boys. They come into puberty on average two years earlier than boys, yet are far more focused on and defined by relationships, and far more concerned about popularity, especially with the opposite sex. At the same time, as we have seen, they lack effective means of influencing males—especially the older boys and young men interested in romantic relationships. Thus, they may find themselves in potentially exploitative or abusive relationships. And, adding to their emotional distress, Frank notes, "this is that point in development at which girls figure out that sexual abuse is wrong."[12]

STAYING SAFE

Societies the world over have traditionally erected strong defenses around their vulnerable young women. Codes of chastity and chivalry, distinctions between "good" and "bad" girls, physical protections ranging from chaperonage to purdah, and elaborate etiquettes of courtship and betrothal all served both to guard girls from male predation and to guide men into commitments providing women security and continuity while raising children. Many of these protective customs—child betrothal, arranged marriages, strict taboos, the cult of virginity, the double standard, rules of exclusion and seclusion, intricate rituals of wooing and affiancing—now appear archaic and demeaning. The advent of safe and reliable contraception has also somewhat evened the sexual balance by lessening the risks of unregulated intercourse.

"Nevertheless," Maccoby insists, "our modern societies, not just America but other industrialized ones, are probably unique in the whole history of human societies in the lack of protection that we provide young women." Unlike traditional systems that build protections into the very fabric of social life, today "the burden of regulating sexuality is placed primarily on young women. There are very few effective taboos left."[13]

And with girls now entering puberty at ages as young as 11, and with the mass media drenching the culture with sexual suggestion, it should come as no surprise that many youngsters find it hard to withstand the new pressures they face. Half of all girls are sexually active by the time they reach 17 and 5 months.[14] Nor should it surprise us that their defenselessness lays girls open to emotional crisis. "Early adversity in the form of childhood sexual abuse, coupled with later adversity in the form of stranger rape, date rape, and other kinds of abuse, along with the apparently universal gender-specific socialization" combine to give girls fewer emotional resources in the face of adversity, Frank believes.[15]

Girls used to confront fewer such dangers. A century ago, menarche came at 15 or so and marriage within the next few years. For her brief season of nubility, a "good" girl could count on community norms to respect and defend her virginity and innocence. Even three decades ago, respectable society held decent men responsible for the consequences of their sexual conduct, even if that required an involuntary trip to the altar.

But the sexual revolution, fueled by the availability of oral contraceptives, changed all that. No single medication has ever had a more sweeping effect on social mores. Nor has any other, among the thousands of tablets and capsules taken by mouth, ever been known simply and universally as the Pill. This epoch-making pharmaceutical fulfilled the ancient dream of freeing women from the fear of unplanned pregnancy and coincided with the demise of the social restraints that used to guard against it.

Today, therefore, although "sexual activity is beginning at younger and younger ages, . . . many girls"—stripped of the protection of now-outdated codes and armed only with persuasive powers relatively ineffective on boys—"are unprepared to handle the pressure from males."[16] But given that the pressures continue, "it shouldn't come as a surprise to us that adolescence is the time at which we begin to see incidence of depression," Maccoby concludes.[17] Sexual abuse is a very real danger to girls of this age.

Most youngsters, of course, still manage a reasonable adjustment during this difficult time. Even so, the years from 14 to 16 constitute another peak age for psychiatric referrals; as many as 10 to 15% of adolescents suffer from a recognizable psychological disorder in any given year. "When adolescents' own reports are taken into account," Conger adds, "the suffering rate is somewhat higher."[18]

In poignant confirmation, each year thousands of youngsters attempt suicide—making an estimated 300 tries for every one that succeeds. Some studies cite figures as high as 20% of American teens, but others offer rather lower rates. Six percent of teenagers queried admitted to a Gallup poll that they had tried at least once. So did 5.6% of the boys and 10.9% of the girls at a school enrolling grades 7 through 12. Fortunately, few of these youthful efforts succeed. Would-be suicides who fall into the category of "attempters"—mostly young females—act impulsively and publicly, using such ineffective means as cutting their wrists. Those in the more dangerous category of "completers"—mostly middle-aged men suffering depression or substance abuse—generally give few warnings, act in private, and use such effective means as hanging or firearms.[19]

Still, this youthful anguish reflects something real: the formidable developmental challenges that lie between puberty and effective adulthood. Adolescents must learn to manage "increased independence from parents, adjustment to sexual maturation, establishment of new and changing workable relationships with peers . . . , deciding about educational and vocational goals, and the development of some sort of basic philosophy of life . . . and a sense of identity," Conger enumerates.[20]

For many girls, success in adolescence entails a contradiction, the necessity of attracting male attention while retaining a satisfactory sense of autonomy and dignity, all the while navigating the treacherous currents of a sexual scene devoid of clear boundaries. A generation or two ago, a "good" girl could safeguard her reputation and hold boys at bay by "playing the field"—dating a number of people, none of whom could claim sufficient intimacy or commitment to demand sexual favors.

In today's much more permissive climate, though, with sexual activity early in a relationship essentially taken for granted, many girls paradoxically feel their "sexual space" much more severely limited than their mothers ever did. They "unwillingly find themselves coerced into exclusive sexual relationships," Maccoby notes. "They don't want to say no entirely and become secluded persons, but they also can't date freely without being considered promiscuous." That venerable defense now implies "the risk of getting a bad reputation. So it's safer for them to hook up with one male who then becomes proprietary." The new sexual "freedom" thus leaves them feeling "coerced and limited."[21]

IN HER OWN IMAGE

This kind of confusion and anxiety over social role and self-image play a major part in many a female adolescence, as a glance at the offerings of any magazine stand makes clear. They also tie directly into all the other big health threats facing teenage girls, smoking, substance abuse, sexually transmitted diseases, pregnancy, and eating disorders. Those at greatest risk for bulimia, for example, "have accepted and internalized most deeply the sociocultural mores of thinness and attractiveness"—the fantastical images of svelte perfection pushed relentlessly by the media— according to Conger.[22]

Bulimia is a subtype of anorexia nervosa, a complex ailment defined by four criteria. Together, they graphically illustrate the close ties among the emotional, physical, and social factors in teens' health. First, the patient refuses to maintain her weight above the minimum normal for her height and age. Second, she (and nearly all anorexics are female) intensely fears gaining weight or becoming fat, despite her actual emacia-tion. Third, she perceives her body's weight and shape inaccurately, be-lieving herself much heavier than she is and denying her serious under-weight. She also gives her weight and figure undue importance in her estimate of her own worth. And finally, starvation has stopped her men-strual periods. Bulimics force down their weight by the potentially deadly cycle of bingeing on food and then making themselves vomit it all up. Other anorexics simply starve themselves, and many exercise intensely to boot.

Given the teen culture's unhealthy emphasis on thinness, "bu-limia unfortunately is a fad," Conger notes, "and occurs frequently, espe-cially on college campuses. Not all people who binge and purge have a psychiatric diagnosis," however. To distinguish mere faddists from the truly disordered, psychiatrists added a final criterion: "A minimum average of two binge eating episodes per week for at least three months."[23]

This frightening condition is "one of the few psychiatric ill-nesses that in and of its own pathology results in death."[24] Sufferers can plunge to a half or even a third of their normal weight. Vomiting can so deplete their bodies' potassium that they go into fatal cardiac arrhythmias. Besides starvation, bulimics die from overdilating their stomachs while bingeing or tearing their esophagus while purging. They take ipecac to induce vomiting, sometimes causing cardiac arrest or irreparable damage that leads to heart failure. Some victims recover—or die—after a single episode. Others relapse and recover again and again. High rates of alcohol and drug abuse and suicide attempts also plague these unfortunate girls.

Anorexia peaks at 14, 15, and 18. "I think this is significant as far as stressors are concerned," Conger says. For "anorectic women who do not appreciate or want to develop a normal female body," the years of blossoming breasts and spreading hips can impose serious stress, Conger notes. Leaving home, as so many 18-year-olds do, seriously stresses girls for whom, as is often the case among anorectics, "dependency is a serious problem."[25] One in 200 girls between 12 and 18 develops anorexia. Ten years later, 6 to 7% of them have died; 30 years later, death has claimed 18 to 21%.[26] Bulimia peaks somewhat later, between 18 and 26 years of age. An estimated 3 to 8% of women between 12 and 40 fall prey, although the death rate is unknown.[27]

The quest for thinness can lead down another path with its own ramifying risks to long-term health. Can it be coincidental, wonders IOM's Committee on Preventing Nicotine Addiction in Children and Youths, that the late 1960s and early 1970s saw a pair of ominous trends? Cigarette companies began targeting certain brands toward young women, explicitly tying tobacco to both fashionable leanness and feminine independence. At the same time, the number of girls under 18 who began smoking "increased abruptly around 1967," topping out "around 1973, at the same time that sales of such brands as Virginia Slims peaked."[28] Ever since the pre-World War II days when ads encouraged them to "Reach for a Lucky instead of a sweet," women have associated lighting up with lightening up. More than 60% of teenage girls who smoke daily and almost half of those who smoke occasionally report, furthermore, that cigarettes calm them.[29] Clearly, emotional stress also works in getting girls to smoke.

As smoking lost its "scarlet woman" image over recent decades, girls have started puffing at earlier and earlier ages. Since 1955, the average age when white girls begin has fallen more than 5 years, to about 12 or 13.[30] (See Table 4-1.) That figure, however, is the only teen smoking statistic that has fallen recently. Adult smoking, on the other hand, declined sharply since the Surgeon General's Report in the mid-1960s; among men alive today, fewer are current than former smokers. Teenage smoking rates also dropped in the 1970s but leveled off in the 1980s.

TABLE 4-1   Percentage of Boys and Girls Who
Initiate Smoking at Specific Ages

Age (years)	Percentage of Age Group	
	Girls	Boys
<9	3.6	6.7
9–10	6.4	8.0
11–12	14.9	16.7
13–14	24.9	24.1
15–16	19.5	19.4
≥17	4.4	5.0

NOTE: Sample sizes for the various age groups were the same (*n* = 11,241) because new smokers who emerged from among those who had never smoked for successive age groups were added incrementally to the numerators of older age groups.

SOURCE: Institute of Medicine, *Growing Up Tobacco Free: Preventing Nicotine Addiction in Children and Youths,* 1994, page 44. Data are from the Youth Risk Behavior Survey, 1990, in Luis G. Escobedo, Stephen Marcus, Deborah Holtzman, and Gary Giovino, "Sports Participation, Age at Smoking Initiation, and the Risk of Smoking among U.S. High School Students." *Journal of the American Medical Association* 17(11):1391–5, 1993.

Between 1992 and 1993, however, experts discerned a small but worrisome rise.[31]

Tobacco advertisers have subtly driven home the notion that smoking smoothes the difficult passage to adult status and sophistication, to popularity and social ease. They also exploit the immaturity of young teens' thinking, which is especially plagued by the difficulty of "envisioning long-term consequences and appreciating the personal relevance of these consequences," notes the nicotine committee. Kids who start smoking, the evidence shows, "do not understand the nature of addiction and, as a result, believe they will be able to avoid" its harmful consequences. "They understand that a lifetime of smoking is dangerous, but they also tend to believe that smoking for a few years will *not* be harmful."[32]

Teens do not generally start out intending to hurt themselves. Still, "adolescent decisions to engage in risky behaviors, including tobacco use, reflect a distinctive focus on short-term benefits and an accompanying tendency to discount long-term risks and dangers," the committee found. Youngsters often "believe that those risks can be controlled by personal choice." In fact, kids usually choose to smoke because they think that large benefits outweigh small risks. "What is most striking, however, is the nature of the trade-off." Reasons for smoking are "transient in nature and closely linked to specific developmental tasks—for example, to assert independence and achieve perceived adult status, or to identify with and establish social bonds with peers who use tobacco."[33] But the results, of course, are potentially permanent—nicotine addiction and its life-shortening risks.

In addition to all the health dangers that cigarettes entail, both for the girl herself and for any children she might bear or raise while a smoker, they expose her to yet another serious peril. Knowing how to smoke serves as the common gateway to the abuse of illicit drugs. No one can use marijuana, crack cocaine, or other smoke-borne drugs who does not know how to inhale smoke.

And once again, the onset of a health-destroying practice relates to young females' complex relationship with males. "Male partners play a critical role in women's initiation and progression in drug use," found IOM's Committee on Substance Abuse and Mental Health Issues in AIDS Research. Males tend to pick up drug use from male friends. For females, though, initiation "occurs most often in the context of love or a sexual relationship or friendship with someone of the opposite sex." Indeed, "having a male partner who uses drugs—especially heavier drug use—places girls at risk of drug use themselves."[34]

The exact extent of teen drug use is not known, in part because surveys tend to study those still in school, a diminishing percentage at the older ages. Both illicit drugs and alcohol are in wide use, however, by boys probably more than by girls. But the female rates of both drinking and drinking to intoxication have been rising faster than the male. Almost 80% of secondary school boys and 70% of girls admit to drinking, one study found, and 23% of boys and 15% of girls to problem drinking. These trends continue upward during the college years. Young people of all ages drink less often than adults, but tend to down much larger amounts when they do.[35]

Alcohol in particular generally carries more severe physical consequences for women than for men. And rather than helping youngsters deal with the emotional burdens of adolescence, mind-altering substances can substantially delay the all-important process of "accomplishing in adolescence the tasks necessary to social maturity," the American School Health Association told an IOM panel. These difficult tasks become even harder "if one's perception of self, time and sequence is distorted or if one's interest or ability in evaluative thinking is impaired."[36] But beyond exposing girls to the dangers of lifetime addiction and physical and mental deterioration, and beyond retarding their own progress toward maturity, and beyond exposing their fetuses to irreparable mental retardation and other defects, substance abuse opens up the very special perils brought on by choices girls make while in a chemical's grip. Injecting drugs carries risks of HIV and other lethal infections. Unprotected sex carries the twin threats of unwanted pregnancy and dangerous, possibly fatal, sexually transmitted diseases.

WAGES OF SEX

Each year, 2.5 million American teens contract sexually transmitted diseases (STDs), running a risk nearly three times that of persons over 20.[37] In addition, nearly 1 million American teens are known to become pregnant each year—fully 1 out of every 10 girls between 15 and 19. Adding in the presumed number of miscarriages raises the total number of conceptions by another 10 to 15%. Every year 470,000 American teens—most of them single, almost half under 18—become mothers. Another 400,000 obtain abortions.[38]

In one statistic at least—rate of teen pregnancies—the U.S. leads all other Western industrial democracies. What explains this sorry distinction? The African American teen pregnancy rate, though considerably higher than the white, does not suffice as an explanation. On their own, and despite a continuing fall in overall adult birth rate, white American teens conceive twice as often as comparable Canadians, citizens of the country closest to our own culturally, geographically, and in terms of pregnancy rates.[39] Americans under 15 are at least 5 times as likely to give birth as girls in any other developed country.[40]

"This disparity is all the more puzzling," notes science writer Suzanne Wymelenberg in an IOM publication, when one considers that "U.S. teenagers are no more sexually active than their peers in similar countries."[41] The answer lies not in sexuality but in society, not in what randy youngsters do, but in what their cultures teach them to do about it. Compared to Sweden, Canada, England and Wales, France, and the Netherlands, American teens make the least use of contraceptives, and when they do use them, they use the least effective kinds. Fewer than half of American girls use any protection at their first intercourse, for example. Of those who do, the condom ranks first, then come the Pill and withdrawal.[42]

This happens in large measure because, compared to other countries, we make it hardest for young people to get birth control. Sweden, the Netherlands, and England and Wales provide services and supplies cheaply or at no charge. The United States does have a national network of family planning clinics that theoretically provide services to teens in most places, but the clinics' historical association with the poor discourages many better-off people from visiting them. Only about 30% of American adolescents get contraceptives from private physicians, discouraged either by the cost or the fear of needing parental permission.[43] Many pediatricians and family doctors, but few gynecologists or obstetricians, admit that they would in fact refuse to prescribe to teens. Nor does Medicaid cover family planning for childless or nonpregnant poor women.

American religious, political, and educational leaders, as well as ordinary citizens, loudly and continually bemoan our nation's dismal record of "children having children." But while their counterparts in other countries "concentrate on preventing teen *pregnancy*," Wymelenberg observes, the American system "concentrates on preventing teen *sex*."[44] Countries that accept both the existence of teen sexuality and the need to provide effective protection against its likely outcome succeed much better than we do in reducing teenage conception.

Properly motivated and properly informed teens, the European experience shows, can successfully contracept. Many conservative French and Dutch physicians initially opposed proposals to provide birth control to teens but changed their opinion when they understood that the alternative was not less adolescent sex but more adolescent abortions. When

Sweden legalized abortion in 1975, the law also made provision for offering birth control to young people, openly acknowledging that, given the realities of teenage behavior, the latter was preferable to the former.

American teenagers, on the other hand, "seem to have inherited the worst of all possible worlds regarding their exposure to messages about sex," note researchers at the Alan Guttmacher Institute, an authority on birth control. "Movies, music, radio and TV tell them that sex is romantic, exciting, titillating; premarital sex and cohabitation are visible ways of life among the adults they see and hear about. . . . Yet, at the same time, young people get the message that good girls should say no. Almost nothing that they see or hear about sex informs them about contraception or the importance of avoiding pregnancy."[45]

Beyond media messages, several other features of American culture and society discourage teens from practicing birth control. Religious communities, which are far more influential in this country than in other Western democracies, often reject not only contraception for teenagers, but even discussions of contraception and sex for teenagers. Our decentralized, locally controlled school system gives such groups greater power than their counterparts have in the centralized, federally controlled educational systems in Europe. Although many people, both within and without the religious community, believe teenage chastity a highly desirable method of preventing youthful pregnancy, experts agree on neither the feasibility of that goal nor the best way of attaining it.

The difficulties that girls have making their wishes known to boys can also contribute, Maccoby believes. Teenage sexual relations are "fraught with possibilities for miscommunication," she observes. "For one thing, it's not uncommon for each member of a pair to expect that the other will take responsibility for contraception. If the young man is more interested in conquest than in protecting the girl, she may find this out too late." Many boys reject condoms as detrimental to pleasure. And, because of their desire for popularity and their weaker skills of persuasion, "many girls will not feel in a position to insist on a boy's using protection if he doesn't volunteer to do it, or, if a girl tries to suggest this, her message may not be received."[46]

Racism, furthermore, keeps many girls in need of contraception from venturing into facilities or neighborhoods perceived as belonging to other groups, as, for example, public family planning clinics thought, because of their locations or predominant clientele, as being "for" African Americans or Hispanic Americans. And the United States permits poverty deeper and more widespread than is tolerated in any other Western industrial democracy. Thus we have a substantial population of hopeless, alienated, poorly educated young people who see no promise of a better future and thus no reason to delay such gratifications as their circumstances afford them. The most potent inoculation against early childbearing may in fact be the hope of a better tomorrow, especially in the form of strong educational goals. African American girls with their sights set on finishing their education are likelier than either white girls or other blacks to use effective forms of contraception.[47]

But even if an American teenager determines to use birth control, she has few options that meet her needs. The most efficacious types, the Pill, the diaphragm, and the intrauterine device, are far better suited to an older woman in a stable, monogamous, predictable sexual relationship than to a young girl whose sexual encounters are likely to be sporadic or unplanned.

To be used successfully, each of these methods requires advance planning and special equipment. Each requires its user to understand—as many youngsters do not—that conception can result from any act of intercourse, even extremely occasional ones, even one's first. And each method, perhaps most importantly from an adolescent's point of view, requires a person to acknowledge to herself and others that she is sexually active, that she is "the kind" of person who both expects to sleep with a man and is willing to make preparations for that eventuality. In a nutshell, it requires her to take responsibility for her sexuality.

In a culture that teaches that "nice girls don't," however, a youngster's self-respect may depend on believing that sex is not something she plans, but only something that occurs spontaneously, in an unpredictable burst of passion. Successfully contracepting requires believing that one has the right and the ability to take active steps to take control of her life. "Adolescent pregnancy could be significantly reduced if a safe, relatively inexpensive, and non-physician-dependent contraceptive were developed for use at the end of the cycles during which intercourse occurs (thereby eliminating the need to plan ahead)," notes Dr. James Trussell, assistant professor of economics and public affairs at Princeton.[48] For reasons we will consider in detail in a later chapter, contraceptive research has slowed to a crawl in the United States. What's more, abortifacients, or substances that cause early abortions, as an "end of the month" pill surely would, remain intensely controversial in a nation still divided over the question of how (or even whether) young girls should be permitted to terminate pregnancies.

A variety of complicated obstacles therefore stand in the way of American attempts to prevent not only teen childbearing but also teen pregnancy. As statistics on falling ages of menarche and smoking and drinking attest, these issues threaten to become more rather than less salient in coming years.

LOOKING FORWARD

The teen years thus occupy a pivotal place in the health of American women. They represent a true crisis, which, in the original Greek meaning, is an event fraught with both danger and opportunity. If a girl can avoid the snares of adolescence, she can look forward to an adulthood free of some of the gravest threats to a long and healthy life.

Almost no one starts smoking or using illicit drugs after age 18 or 20, for example. Avoiding sexually transmitted diseases will safeguard both her fertility and her life. Delaying her first child until her mid-twenties vastly reduces her chances of spending her life in poverty (delaying much longer than that, however, somewhat raises her risk of breast cancer). Eating a sound, high-calcium diet and developing the habit of regular exercise will help prevent cardiovascular disorders, the largest killer of women; reproductive cancers; and osteoporosis. Risk of this last disease depends so significantly on the quantity of bone a woman builds up in her adolescence and twenties that, as Charles Chestnut of the National Osteoporosis Foundation notes, this impairment of old age "may be a pediatric disease," whose solution lies in the teen years.[49]

But, he goes on, "it is obviously very difficult for young women aged 15 to be concerned about a disease that may occur 40 years later,"[50] or, even, as experience with teens indicates, to be concerned about dangers that lie a day or a week or a month away. For too many American girls, a turbulent adolescence lays the foundation not for a lifetime of good health but for later bouts of avoidable disorders, both physical and emotional. We will watch these forces play out in the chapters that follow.

NOTES

1. *Research on Children and Adolescents with Mental, Behavioral, and Developmental Disorders: Mobilizing a National Initiative*, 73.
2. Ibid., 74.
3. Assessing Future Research Needs: Mental and Addictive Disorders in Women (Transcript), 177.
4. IOM 1992 Annual Meeting, 126.
5. Assessing Future Research Needs (Transcript), 151.
6. Ibid., 142.
7. Ibid.
8. Ibid., 143.
9. Ibid., 154-5.
10. IOM 1992 Annual Meeting, 126.
11. Assessing Future Research Needs (Transcript), 148.
12. IOM 1992 Annual Meeting, 126.
13. Assessing Future Research Needs (Transcript), 149.
14. Forrest (1991), 4.
15. IOM 1992 Annual Meeting, 128.
16. Assessing Future Research Needs (Transcript), 149.
17. Ibid., 150.
18. Ibid., 152.
19. Ibid., 192-3.
20. Ibid., 151.
21. Ibid., 149.
22. Ibid., 158.
23. Ibid., 209.
24. Ibid., 210.
25. Ibid., 211.
26. Ibid.
27. Ibid., 212.
28. *Growing Up Tobacco Free: Preventing Nicotine Addiction in Children and Youths*, 116.
29. Ibid., 49.
30. Ibid., 106.
31. Ibid., 8.
32. Ibid., 14.
33. Ibid., 15.
34. *AIDS and Behavior: An Integrated Approach*, 96.
35. *Health and Behavior: Frontiers of Research in the Biobehavioral Sciences*, 248.
36. *Healthy People 2000: Citizens Chart the Course*, 105-6.
37. Ibid., 159.
38. Ibid.
39. *Science and Babies: Private Decisions, Public Dilemmas*, 70-1.
40. Ibid., 8.
41. Ibid., 70.

42. Ibid., 57.
43. Ibid., 71.
44. Ibid., 88.
45. Quoted ibid.
46. IOM 1992 Annual Meeting, 88-9.
47. *Science and Babies*, 76.
48. Quoted ibid., 91.
49. Quoted in *Healthy People 2000*, 197.
50. Quoted ibid.

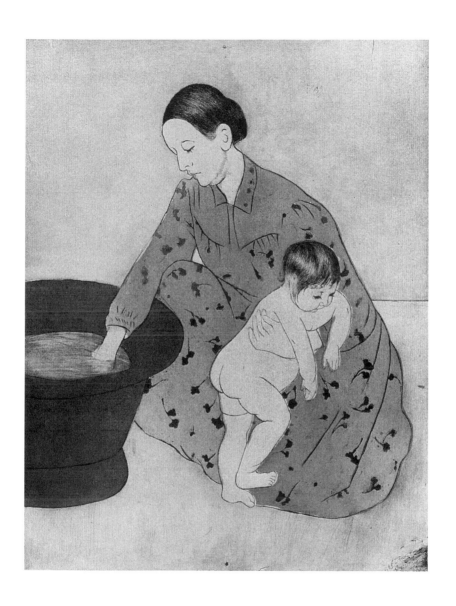

Mary Cassatt
The Bath (1891)
Soft-ground etching with aquatint and drypoint on paper
The National Museum of Women in the Arts
Gift of Wallace and Wilhelmina Holladay

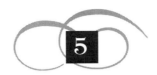

Health Through the
Life Span:
The Reproductive Years

No single event marks the threshold to American adulthood. In many traditional societies, on the other hand, the transition to the status of the fully grown (and fully responsible) adult happens abruptly and in public. Rituals recognizing the onset of menstruation, or the attainment of a certain age, or the successful completion of prescribed tasks or trials, or initiation into a secret society, or any of a number of other milestones, have for millennia ushered junior members into manhood or womanhood. Even within living American memory, the formal debut transformed upper-class schoolgirls into marriageable women in a whirl of balls and tea dances. Mere generations ago, an American boy graduated into long pants and an American girl put up her hair and dropped her hemline to mark the passage to man's and woman's estate.

But today Americans generally osmose into adulthood, taking on the prerogatives of their majority only by gradual, and often confusing, degrees. We can generally drive, drop out of school, and get a regular job at 16. Most people, though, continue their studies at least through high school graduation at about 18, the age that allows voting, military service, and signing valid contracts. But no one can legally drink until 21, and various states permit marriage at various ages, often different for the two sexes. Nor does any one of these conflicting milestones in itself confer universally recognized maturity.

The cost of post-secondary education often further delays entree to adulthood, keeping many people dependent on their families well into their twenties. A tight employment market can do the same, forcing large numbers back into their parents' homes even after earning degrees or credentials that theoretically equip them to make their own way. Meanwhile, as they pass all these formal landmarks, American youth, as we have seen, also traverse, each at his or her own pace, an informal curriculum of adult behaviors that includes initiation into sexual activity, and, for far too many, into smoking, drinking, and drug use as well.

At various points, young people also pass from the medical care arrangements that saw them through their growing-up years, either outgrowing their pediatricians or moving away to campus, military posting, or out-of-town work. Depending on their own and their families' financial, employment, and educational situations, they also eventually lose coverage under their parents' health insurance. What, if anything, replaces it depends on each individual's eligibility in his or her own right to benefits from the military, student health services, employers' insurance plans, or public assistance programs.

For most Americans, fortunately, this period of awkward transition is also an era of excellent health. The childhood ailments are over, and the commonest chronic diseases and debilities lie decades in the future. Only violence and accidents, usually involving firearms or motor vehicles, claim substantial numbers of young lives, more often male than female.

A MAJOR CHALLENGE

This does not mean, however, that women entering or even well into their third decade have no serious health needs. For the overwhelming majority, sexual activity, whether within or without marriage, has become a routine and open fact of life. For at least the next two decades, fertility and its consequences dominate most women's health—as well as economic, social, and career—concerns.

For women, of course, the issue of when and whether to have

children, and then whether and how to raise them, shapes not only physical well-being, but also personal identity, career prospects, and, to a large extent, economic status. The fact, indeed, that childbearing is now an issue, rather than, as it was for millennia, an unavoidable and generally uncontrollable fact of life, indicates the immense importance of the technologies that now allow women largely to shape, rather than merely to endure, their reproductive destinies.

The three decades since the introduction of modern contraception (which also subsume the two decades since *Roe v. Wade* overturned almost all bans on elective abortion) have seen perhaps the most drastic change in gender roles and attitudes in human history. Women on aircraft carriers, construction sites, and the Supreme Court; women as army generals, attorneys general, and surgeons general; women outnumbering men in newsrooms, elite medical schools, manufacturing plants; women entering every occupation from astronaut to zookeeper—this social revolution closely followed two other revolutions, the technological one that culminated in the Pill and the judicial one that legalized abortion.

It might seem, then, that the miracle of modern medicine has essentially resolved American women's reproductive dilemma, reducing it to a mere personal decision about when most conveniently to have one's desired number of planned children. For millions, though, this complacent assumption is far from the truth. Despite their huge strides in the workplace, American women trying to control their fertility face an increasingly difficult situation.

"Since 1980 the reproductive health status of Americans has deteriorated," Wymelenberg writes for IOM. "The rates of unintended pregnancy and abortion in the United States are among the highest in the Western world, and our rates for adolescent pregnancy, abortion and childbearing are the highest. In infant mortality, a key indicator of national health, the United States ranks twentieth among industrialized nations, behind Hong Kong and Singapore. Despite our considerable research resources, American women have fewer contraceptive choices than their European counterparts. More than half the 6 million pregnancies that occur annually in this country are unintended, and half those unintended pregnancies—about 1.6 million—end in abortion. Meanwhile, concern about infertility appears to be increasing among many men and women."[1]

A sharp dichotomy between millions who find themselves unwillingly pregnant and countless others who long vainly to conceive hardly indicates a nation in control of its fertility. The spectacle, furthermore, of thousands of newborns needlessly suffering and dying from preventable problems seems alien to a nation blessed with the best in medical resources the world has ever known. And yet the same United States that suffers these ills also gave the world both the Pill and the IUD and has long been at the forefront of both science and practice in obstetrics and pediatrics. As we will explore in later chapters, features of our health care delivery and research systems in large measure account for these medical anomalies.

The vast majority of American women and couples seeking the right contraceptive strategy to limit their fertility in fact face a daunting problem even apart from macroscale issues of social structure. Over 95% of the nation's more than 54 million sexually experienced women of childbearing age also have at least some experience with contraception. Over 70% of the married couples in the fertile years use some form of birth control. The Pill is the nation's popular choice, followed by female sterilization, condoms, and male sterilization. "Never before in history," notes IOM's Committee on Contraception about the choice made by one-third of the women at risk for unintended pregnancy, "has a systemic drug such as the oral contraceptive been used so widely on a continuing basis by predominantly healthy women for a protective purpose."[2]

But the list of choices open to Americans also goes a long way to explaining some puzzling disparities. Only one of the leading methods would seem to meet most people's criteria for a highly desirable contraceptive; only one, in other words, is very effective, takes advantage of advanced research, does not impinge on the sexual act, and allows people to change their minds and later become pregnant. And that one, the Pill, requires daily attention and raises safety issues for some individuals. Of the other leading choices, the condom—used by 16% of the partners of women who face unintended pregnancy—is a crude and ancient device that requires discipline, interferes with pleasure, and depends for its effectiveness on users paying meticulous attention every single time. The remaining two options demand a surgical operation as well as a usually irreversible decision never again to have children.

Despite this often dismaying finality, sterilization is still the preference of one-fifth of all the women between 18 and 49 at risk for unintentional pregnancy and 15% of their male partners.[3] Indeed, "fifteen or more years after their first marriage," the committee notes, "44% of all women practicing contraception are sterilized, and another 24% are married to men who are sterilized."[4] Why so many more women than men take this step, despite the greater difficulty and danger of the female procedure, probably involves both differences in the strength of one's desire not to conceive and differing notions of manhood and womanhood. Still, between 2 and 13% of women—especially those sterilized in their twenties or early thirties—regret their decision within 6 months to 6 years. As many as 8% seek to reverse the operation surgically, but only a minority of these attempts succeed.[5]

A DEARTH OF OPTIONS

These figures, along with the problems that we have already seen facing teenagers who seek suitable contraception, certainly suggest that many Americans have contraceptive needs unmet by any available option. There are only four other readily available possibilities: withdrawal and abstinence, the choice of 5% each; the diaphragm, used by 4 to 6%; the IUD, the choice of 3%; and foams, jellies, creams, and suppositories, at about 1% each.[6] A new category of long-lasting contraceptives, the subdermal (under-skin) implants, involve placing a unit under the skin to provide a continuing supply of hormonal medication not unlike that found in the Pill. They are highly reliable and protect for months or years at a time, but have thus far been used in this country only on a very limited scale.

Like the Pill, the condom, and sterilization, moreover, each of these reversible methods has serious faults for at least some users. The diaphragm and IUD are generally quite safe and effective (and, in the case of the diaphragm, provide some protection from infection), but both require doctor visits and medical supervision that place them beyond the means of some people. The diaphragm must be correctly inserted each time and later removed for cleaning, requirements that many find intrusive and unaesthetic. The IUD is not suitable for young women before a first birth. The remaining popular methods, though cheap and easily used without a prescription, are markedly less reliable. The implants require minor surgery for both installation and removal.

In short, "every method in use today has drawbacks," the committee concludes, "and collectively, current methods leave major gaps in the ability of people to control fertility safely, effectively, and in culturally acceptable ways throughout their reproductive life cycle."[7] Americans face widely varying, and often changing, circumstances. Successful birth control requires contraceptives tailored to the individual's particular needs. As we have seen, teenagers face one set of problems in finding a method that works, and women in other circumstances face different, but equally troubling, obstacles. For example, low-income Hispanic women, concluded Scrimshaw and colleagues in a Los Angeles study, have no acceptable method that allows them both to breastfeed and reliably to space their families. They fear the Pill may interfere with lactation, and they reject barrier methods as unsuitable either for their partners or themselves. The IUD has no effect on breastfeeding but does have a high propensity to fail, be expelled, or perforate the uterus when inserted shortly after birth.[8] Possible hormonal effects of implants on nursing babies are not known.

Advancing age and special health needs also form obstacles to using some of the most reliable methods. The Pill, for example, is less safe for women over 35 or who smoke. Neither hormonal nor intrauterine methods suit those with insulin-dependent diabetes or those with certain cardiovascular conditions; both categories need contraception that neither aggravates their diseases nor raises their risk of infection.

And even if a woman is physically suited to a method, her circumstances and skills may not permit her to use it to best advantage. Studies of various developed and developing countries have shown that not all groups, even within the same nation, can use all methods with equal effectiveness. Educated women and those who have all the children they want generally enjoy the greatest success.[9]

A couple's chances of avoiding pregnancy depend, moreover, not only on their motivation and knowledge but also on the method they choose. Better than 99.5% of sterilized men and women, for example, can rest assured that they will not conceive in the first year after the operation. The same goes for 97% of Pill users and 94% of IUD users. Only 88% of condom users, will succeed, however, and 82% of those depending on the diaphragm, cervical cap, or withdrawal. Fewer than four-fifths of those counting on periodic abstinence, the contraceptive sponge, or spermicidal creams and jellies used alone will find their faith justified.[10]

Even though success rates of the various methods tend to rise in subsequent years as users become more expert at using them, the failure rates represent large numbers of lives disrupted by unplanned pregnancies. The average 8% failure rate of the condom, for example (a number that includes both new and experienced users), represents more than half a million American women facing pregnancies they did not intend. In all, contraceptive failure accounts for between 1.6 and 2 million such "accidents" each year, and about three quarters of a million abortions.[11] These failures, plus the fact that many women spend substantial periods of time without the protection of an appropriate method, add up to unintended pregnancy for more than half of American women at some time in their lives.[12] "We could reduce abortions in this country by 50% overnight if we had totally successful contraception," says Sheldon Segal, Ph.D., distinguished scientist at the Population Council in New York.[13]

"One polio vaccine solved the problem of poliomyelitis," the contraceptive committee observes, "but one contraceptive will never meet all societies' and all individuals' changing needs. . . . There are important and obvious gaps in the range of available methods. These gaps could be filled, in part, by developing new, safe, effective and acceptable methods for men, for breastfeeding women, for teenagers, for older women, and for those with particular health conditions."[14]

Far from welcoming exciting innovations to the market, though, the American public has actually seen contraceptive options contract in recent years, as manufacturers have withdrawn products, particularly IUDs, from sale in this country in the wake of the Dalkon Shield disaster, in which a combination of faulty design and corporate duplicity injured scores of thousands of women and resulted in a financial settlement in excess of $2 billion.

In addition, "since the introduction of the pill and the IUD in the early 1960s, no fundamentally new contraceptive methods have been approved for use in the United States," the committee notes, although several have become available abroad. Nor does it foresee "dramatic changes" in the years ahead. Although various lines of inquiry may eventually yield useful results, "one person's promising new development is, for another, a preposterous idea or only a trivial modification."[15]

Our nation's relatively dismal contraceptive record cannot be attributed only to lack of methods. Countries that do better than we do in preventing unwanted pregnancies also do better at getting existing products into the hands of those who need them. In this country, most women consult obstetricians and gynecologists for contraceptive care; in the more successful countries, family doctors generally provide this service. Here family planning clinics serve those who cannot afford a private physician; in the more successful countries, they specialize in counseling first-time users of many social classes. Here "the choice of a caregiver is determined by the patient's financial state; in other countries, the determinant is the patient's need," Wymelenberg notes.[16] Contraceptives are costly in the United States, but elsewhere they are cheap or free. In other countries, advertising, education, publicity, even brochures distributed in drugstores, spread information about sexuality and birth control. In this country, the mass media give low priority to informing the public about contraception. Many schools, too, are constrained in the instruction they offer.

This information gap leaves the young and poorly educated largely ignorant of the true risks of unprotected intercourse and the real advantages of effective contraception. It also leaves unchallenged many women's unfounded fears about safety. More than three-quarters of American women, for example, believe that oral contraceptives carry substantial health risks. In fact, however, three times as many Americans—14 per 100,000—die each year in childbirth as die from the Pill. Besides being much safer than carrying to term for the woman under 35 who smokes fewer than 15 cigarettes daily, it also protects against cancer of the endometrium and ovaries, benign breast tumors, ectopic pregnancy and pelvic inflammatory disease—advantages that outweigh any cardiovascular risk it may carry.[17]

TERMINATING PREGNANCIES

"When a contraceptive fails, whether the man or woman was using it, the health of the woman is put at risk," Segal says.[18] Our nation's high abortion rate clearly mirrors our outsized rate of unwanted pregnancy, and in both of these dubious distinctions we lead the Western industrial democracies. What distinguishes us is not our level of sexual activity, which varies little among the Westernized countries, but two other equally dubious world records: the low availability of the most effective means of controlling the outcome of that activity, especially the Pill; and the highest percentage of women using no contraception of any developed nation.[19] With 28.5 abortions per 1,000 women per year, we outpace the Netherlands by 500% and rank about midway among the nations that keep accurate abortion statistics, close to Singapore and the former East Germany. On average, American couples want 1.25 children but end up instead with 1.6 kids and an abortion.[20]

For that procedure, most American women choose first trimester vacuum aspiration, a minor surgical procedure. Later terminations re quire more complicated interventions. All the methods available here can require a woman to wait, sometimes for several weeks, between the discovery of the pregnancy and the point when it can be safely and effectively terminated. As with contraception, many authorities argue, Americans need a wider range of choices.

Any new techniques, however, must consider "both moral and physiological ideals, as well as psychological concerns," states Étienne-Émile Baulieu, M.D., Ph.D., of the Faculté de Médecine Paris-sud in France. "For centuries, abortion has been not only a morally difficult event for women, but also a physically painful and often dangerous procedure." Thus, any "medical means for pregnancy termination should diminish this threat to women's health" as well as "allow them to maintain their dignity."[21]

What's more, "the beginning of pregnancy is now understood to be a progression of steps" rather than a single event as formerly thought. Physicians and lay people had once believed that the moment when a woman first felt her fetus move, an event traditionally known as the "quickening" (literally "coming to life"), marked the actual change of a previously inert mass into a living creature. Today we know that two gametes merge into a single-celled being that multiplies, travels, embeds itself in the womb, changes form, and grows into a person able to live outside the mother's body through a number of stages separated by no sharp breaks. This process can therefore be halted at a number of points both before and after fertilization. Thus, "the distinction between abortion and contraception has lessened," Baulieu notes.[22]

In light of all these issues, "to develop a medical [as opposed to a surgical] method was a must in terms of women's health and potentially a step toward more privacy for those having taken the difficult decision of pregnancy termination."[23] Baulieu and others thus sought a method "that can provoke pregnancy interruption . . . as soon as possible after pregnancy has occurred, before the word abortion is appropriate."[24] In addition, they wanted something "safer than surgical technique" and "relatively convenient and cheap (no anesthesia, no operating room)."[25]

The drug mifepristone, more commonly know as RU 486, fulfilled these requirements so strikingly that it "immediately got the nickname 'abortion pill,' despite the many other potential medical uses already predicted when the compound was announced" and which ultimately came to realization.[26] Given along with the compound prostaglandin, it counteracts the body's own progesterone, a hormone essential to maintaining early pregnancy. "Almost a decade of research is now available" on this action by RU 486, notes the IOM's Committee on Antiprogestins (the technical name for this class of drugs). "Drug regulatory officials in France, Sweden and the United Kingdom" have found it a "safe and efficacious medical treatment for early pregnancy termination."[27]

But not, as yet, in the United States, where the controversy over abortion created a climate that discouraged the French manufacturer, Roussel-Uclaf, from entering the U.S. market. In an April 1993 Executive Order, President Clinton called for research into uses of the antiprogestins. With RU 486 now licensed by Roussel to the Population Council, an American nonprofit organization, FDA approval is anticipated in 1997.

"As a pharmacological class, the antiprogestins appear to have great potential as regulators of reproductive potential," the committee continues.[28] In addition to facilitating first trimester abortions, possibilities include use as a "morning-after pill," to provide retroactive contraceptive protection; and to promote cervical ripening, whether for late-trimester abortions, termination of dead fetuses, or induced deliveries at full term. Much broader uses also wait to be explored, including promising leads in treating endometriosis; fibroid tumors of the uterus; breast cancer; tumors of the membranes around the brain; and Cushing's syndrome, a disease of the adrenal gland.

INFERTILITY

While the fear of unwanted pregnancy bedevils tens of millions of Americans, other millions struggle with the opposite problem: inability to conceive or bear children when they wish—or, in many cases, ardently crave—to. Doctors consider a couple infertile if they do not conceive in a year of unprotected intercourse or if they do conceive but cannot carry a baby to term. At least 2.3 million married couples—1 in every 12 in the nation—experience this frustration. The overall infertility rate has fallen somewhat in the last 30 years, most markedly among families that already have at least one child and desire more (a condition known as secondary infertility).[29]

The same period, however, has seen almost a doubling of young women unable to have a first child. At least 7% of 20- to 24-year-olds, the group that bears a third of all babies born in this country, now suffer from this so-called primary infertility, mainly because diseases like gonorrhea and chlamydia are so widespread among today's sexually very active young people. Infections often picked up—and possibly even discovered, treated, and cured—in adolescence or the very early years of adulthood thus can leave lifelong physical and psychological scars. Second only to the common cold and influenza in frequency, these two diseases account for almost 40% of infertility in this country.[30] The total number of involuntarily childless couples has also doubled since 1965 to 1 million.[31]

Ninety percent of infertility arises from some cause that doctors can pinpoint, and half of couples receiving fertility treatment do succeed in conceiving at least once. Most of those go on to have a child.[32] The hunt for an answer generally starts with the woman's doctor, either a family practitioner or a gynecologist, the specialty that does about 80% of basic infertility treatment.[33] A urologist usually checks the man for problems. If these efforts do not produce results, the quest often leads next to physicians, practices, or clinics specializing in infertility, frequently highly expert teams at medical schools or major hospital centers.

Because, as we have noted, a pregnancy can be prevented or stopped at many points, a large number of causes, or a combination of causes, may account for any specific case. As each is painstakingly eliminated, the "infertility workup" can become a costly, draining, and onerous experience. Female problems can include adhesions, the scars that can result from infections or surgery, which block or interfere with the delicate workings of the fallopian tubes and other organs; problems with ovulation; and endometriosis, the growth of the cells that normally line the uterus in other, inappropriate parts of the body.

On the male side, inadequately numerous or vigorous sperm are the main problem, caused by a variety of factors, including varicoceles, or dilations of testicular blood vessels; and damage to passages or organs from infection. Infertility research to date has concentrated mostly on the female system. Despite progress in recent years, "more needs to be known about the reproductive physiology of the male and about diagnosing and treating sperm deficiencies," Wymelenberg notes, as well as "the basic process of sperm movement through the female reproductive tract."[34]

Fertility treatment ranges from something as simple as determining the likely time of ovulation to immensely sophisticated in vitro fertilization (IVF) procedures. They may include surgery for varicoceles, which succeeds about three times in four; hormonal interventions to improve ovulation, successful about half the time; artificial insemination, with about a one-third success rate; and surgery to correct fallopian or uterine deformities, whose success varies widely, depending on the exact condition and the surgeon's skill. In any procedure using donated semen, the Centers for Disease Control and Prevention strongly suggests that the donor's blood be tested for HIV both at the time of donation and six months later. In the meantime, to guard against possible infection, the waiting semen should be frozen and quarantined while in storage.[35]

Beyond these treatments lies the frontier of truly high-tech reproductive medicine, IVF and the newer techniques based on it, such as gamete interfallopian transfer (GIFT). In 1978, after decades of research, the first "test-tube" baby, Louise Brown, was born in England to worldwide headlines. From a science fiction fantasy, these methods have now become the basis of a rapidly growing and largely unregulated multibillion-dollar industry. From a single clinic in the Oldham and District Hospital in Lancashire, they have spread to hundreds of facilities around the world.

Used as a last resort when simpler methods do not suffice—particularly in cases of missing or blocked fallopian tubes, female antibodies against the sperm, endometriosis, and other problems that prevent normal transport of egg and sperm—these high-tech methods require a panoply of difficult and sophisticated procedures, including manipulations of hormones, ripening and harvesting of eggs, and their reintroduction into the woman's body. In IVF, actual fertilization takes place "in vitro"—literally, "in glass"—but on a laboratory dish rather than in the proverbial test tube. In GIFT, which is possible if the woman has a functional fallopian tube, recovered eggs are deposited, along with sperm, in the tube, in hopes that fertilization will proceed normally from there on.

Such delicate and demanding maneuvers obviously require extreme skill and excellent facilities, which equally obviously add up to very considerable cost. Each single attempt runs at least several thousand dollars, and because the success rate for any given attempt is well below 20%, many couples try numerous times before either succeeding or giving up. What constitutes "success," furthermore, is a subject of some controversy. Some facilities, in publicizing their services, claim that accolade whenever a pregnancy occurs, whether or not it results in a live birth—and many such "successes" do not. Because a federal ban on fetal research long prohibited any government participation in IVF and related techniques at either the laboratory or the clinical level, government oversight has also been largely absent from a specialty financed primarily by patients' private fees and fueled by the often desperate and sometimes unrealistic hopes of couples unable to fulfill a deeply held desire.

Insurance coverage for fertility treatments varies, but rarely picks up anything close to the full fee. "Current costs for infertility treatments are so substantial that they place infertility care beyond the reach of low-income couples, and they represent a sizable investment for middle-income couples," Wymelenberg observes. Indeed, infertility patients come disproportionately from the well-off and well-educated. Though African Americans suffer infertility half again as often as whites, they seek treatment less often. Hundreds of thousands of Americans with primary infertility, in fact, have never even sought help. One study estimated that a couple earning under $20,000 a year could incur out-of-pocket bills representing 62% of their annual income for typical treatment regimens—and that assumes that they have health insurance, an increasingly tenuous assumption for people in all income brackets. Even an insured couple earning over $35,000 could spend 12% or more or their income.[36] Most states, furthermore, forbid Medicaid reimbursement for treatments to enhance fertility.

Given these extremely high costs and often disappointingly low success rates, not to mention the physical and emotional stress of complicated and sometimes painful tests, as well as the anxiety and discomfort of often extremely intrusive treatments, Americans badly need a wider choice of more reliable solutions to this increasingly common problem.

PREGNANCY AND BIRTH

Despite American women's struggles to limit or enhance their fertility, the great majority, do, of course, at some point bear children. But the statistics describing the fate of our nation's newborns, like those concerning unwanted pregnancy, infertility, and abortion, indicate that this country, though possessing a concentration of medical talent, knowledge and resources unmatched in the history of the world, fails to afford to many of its citizens the simple, basic health services that can make a huge difference at an utterly crucial point in their lives. The plain fact is that we rank very near the bottom of the industrialized democracies in the most essential indicator of maternal and neonatal well-being, the infant mortality rate.

In 1918, we ranked sixth among 20 selected countries.[37] Sixty years later, our undistinguished though still respectable standing remained essentially unchanged. In the 1980s, however, it began to drop sharply, plummeting to nineteenth place by the end of the decade, behind such countries as Hong Kong, Singapore, and Spain.[38] At more than 10 per 1,000 births, our average national newborn mortality rate exceeds those three countries' by more than 10% and those of the top-ranking countries, Japan, Finland, and Sweden, by almost 170%.[39] Even more shockingly,

African American infant death rates in some of our states exceed 20 per 1,000. For the nation as a whole, they average 18 per 1,000, about twice the white rate of between 8 and 11 per 1,000, and three times the 6 per 1,000 attained by the leading countries.[40]

The cause of this appalling performance is not in the least mysterious: more than 10% of American babies are born weighing abnormally little for their gestational age, many of them premature.[41] The traditional line on birth announcements noting the infant's weight represents more than an amusing bit of trivia. That figure is perhaps the single best indicator of the child's well-being and immediate prospects for survival. Entering the world at less than 5 pounds, 8 ounces (2,500 grams) places a child in the problematic category of low birth weight; and at less than 3 pounds, 5 ounces (1,500 grams) in the quite perilous one of very low birth weight.[42]

A baby born underweight, whatever the cause, lacks the benefit of adequate fetal growth and emerges from the engulfing nurturance of the womb less than optimally equipped to face the challenges of the air-breathing, mouth-feeding, microbe-infested outer world. The farther he falls below the norm, the greater his risk of early death or, if he survives, of serious, possibly lifelong, complications.

Nor is the cause of low birth weight hard to discern. It results primarily from inadequate or nonexistent prenatal care. Getting good-quality, consistent medical attention from the early months of pregnancy can make a crucial difference in a child's chances of being born at the right time and weight. A baby whose mother lacks such care faces five times the risk of death as one whose mother received it. With a proper regime of examinations and counseling, health professionals can discover and treat many of the conditions that can complicate the pregnancy or compromise the fetus. They can also advise the mother on diet; level of rest and activity; abstinence from tobacco, drugs, and alcohol; care with medications; and other lifestyle factors that can maximize both her own and her baby's welfare.

On the basis of examining 55 studies of factors affecting infant health, the Congressional Office of Technology Assessment concluded that the evidence "supports the contention that two key birth outcomes—low birth weight and neonatal mortality—can be improved with earlier and more comprehensive prenatal care, especially in high-risk groups such as adolescents and the poor."[43] It also contributes to the mother's own chances of surviving delivery. Maternal deaths often result from pregnancies that implant in the fallopian tubes rather than the uterus (ectopic pregnancies), and miscarriages that involve infections (septic abortions).[44] Astonishingly, in this age of everyday medical marvels, more than three times as many African American women die from maternal causes as whites, a discrepancy probably "due to minority women's lack of access to, or underutilization of, obstetrical services," says the IOM's Committee on Health Objectives for the Year 2000. Proper care could save three-quarters of those lives.[45]

Slightly fewer than 70% of all Americans get adequate prenatal care—"nearly three-quarters of white women but only one-half of black women," IOM's Committee on Monitoring Access to Personal Health Care Services found, citing figures from the late 1980s. Just three-quarters of all pregnant Americans got medical attention in the first trimester— 80% of whites, over 86% of Japanese Americans, but only 60% of African Americans and even fewer Native Americans and Mexican Americans— with the racial discrepancies worsening in the 1980s.[46] In those same years, most teenage African American mothers had no first trimester care at all. Fully 14% of these young women either got no medical attention before the last trimester or went to term without ever getting any.[47]

It is clearly not accidental that these figures coincide with the plunge in our nation's standing relative to comparable countries. Nor, as we will explore in a later chapter, are they unrelated to other complex legal and medical issues bedeviling our health care system.

This country, meanwhile, countenances spending tens of thousands of dollars for infertility treatments and hundreds of thousands for high-tech rescues of grossly underweight and premature infants while many expectant mothers cannot obtain a couple of thousand dollars of preventative care that would help promote the safe delivery of a healthy child. If the nation increased access to prenatal care enough to reduce our rate of low birth weight by 2.5%, an IOM study found, our health care system could save $3 on later treatment of underweight infants for every $1 spent treating pregnant mothers.[48] Indeed, infant mortality did drop by two-thirds between 1965 and 1980 before leveling off. Few of those lives were saved by relatively cheap measures to raise birth weight, however. Most involved the drama and high cost of neonatal intensive care, which has dramatically, if expensively, improved its ability to rescue tiny, highly vulnerable newborns.[49]

When the time comes for a woman to deliver, American medicine again shows its penchant for expensive high-tech interventions rather than cheaper and simpler alternatives. About one American baby in four arrives by cesarean section, the world's highest rate. Women over 30 are two or three times likelier than others to deliver by cesarean, and privately insured patients and those with private doctors also do so more often than others.[50] Today's cesarean rate also substantially exceeds that customary in this country only a generation ago.[51] As recently as 1965, it was under 5% of births. Since then, failure to progress in labor, breech presentation, and fetal distress—all conditions commonly diagnosed with electronic fetal monitoring—have become common reasons for resorting to cesarean. Nearly half of all cesareans, however, were performed because the mother had the procedure for a previous delivery.[52]

For almost 100 years, American physicians have followed the dictum of E.B. Cragin, M.D., chairman of obstetrics and gynecology at Columbia University's prestigious College of Physicians and Surgeons: "Once a cesarean, always a cesarean." In Cragin's day, this rule made good sense, because the scar formed by the so-called classical cesarean section, a vertical incision of the uterus, had a high tendency to rupture during the strain of subsequent labor. Since then, however, a cesarean technique involving a lower, horizontal incision much less subject to later rupture has come into wide use. Research has shown that women who have had that procedure can safely try vaginal delivery for later births, and that the great majority of them can successfully deliver vaginally.[53] Indeed, the American College of Obstetricians and Gynecologists, which encourages this approach, has issued guidelines for deciding who is eligible.

Though the cesarean does improve survival chances of very small, high-risk babies and those presenting by the breech, this costly procedure is far more difficult and dangerous for the mother, exposing her to major abdominal surgery with its risks of infection and other complications.[54] But the decision to use it may involve, as we will discuss in detail in a later chapter, reasons that have as much to do with the welfare of insurance companies as of women and infants.

Whether women delivering by cesarean make a more difficult transition to motherhood than those who deliver vaginally is not clear. It is obvious, however, that many women, no matter how they delivered, do find this major life passage quite stressful. Some 10% suffer a depression following childbirth that is severe enough to interfere with their daily lives.[55] This so-called postpartum depression can involve either unipolar or bipolar disorder. Though most of these depressive episodes pass quickly, some last as long as two years. And even after their depression lifts, some new mothers continue to have difficulty with mood. Women who have not suffered other depressions unrelated to childbirth seem to have the best chance of full recovery.[56]

MENTAL DISORDERS

Depression, whether technically "postpartum" or not, is a much greater problem for women than for men during the reproductive years, notes the IOM's Committee on Health and Behavior, and most "particularly for mothers and young wives."[57] Is it biochemistry or bawling babies that afflicts them? Like puberty, the era of early marriage and young children combines rapid hormonal changes with drastic and often abrupt transformations of a woman's self-image and expectations. Once again we are left to ponder the relative contributions of hormones and the stress of trying to fulfill demanding and often conflicting roles. With many mothers holding down tiring jobs both inside and outside the home, with high-quality child care still an expensive and hard-to-find necessity, with growing numbers of women raising children on their own, the sources of depression, anxiety, substance abuse, and other mental disorders present little mystery.

Among adults, alcohol is the most common drug of abuse, although the binge drinking of youth drops off for both genders as people take on the responsibilities of adulthood. Marriage in particular seems to have a sobering effect. "In the aggregate," remarks Kaye Fillmore, Ph.D., of the Institute for Health and Aging at the University of California San Francisco, "men and women seem to waltz or foxtrot or jitterbug across the life course in tandem by age with respect to their main drinking patterns." When one gender's average intake increases or decreases, so does the other's. At no point, however, does "women's drinking level exceed that of the men's."[58] In particular, women between 25 and 34 generally drink quite moderately, a finding that holds across "culture and history," Fillmore adds, "suggesting the influence of childbearing and childrearing."[59]

Some women do, however, either begin or continue drinking to excess. An important precipitant appears to be divorce. For reasons still not entirely understood, furthermore, the number of young women in alcohol treatment programs has risen noticeably in the past 15 years. About a third of Alcoholics Anonymous members are now female, a rise over former years, when the fellowship was overwhelmingly male. Even so, experts believe women are still underrepresented in treatment; twice as many males as females appear to abuse alcohol, but four times as many come forward to seek treatment. A stigma much stronger than that for men, including an ancient association of female drunkenness with loose sexuality, seems to keep many women from coming forward for help.[60]

Still, chemically dependent women need treatment as much as men, and possibly more. As we have already noted, many more females than males suffer severe depression along with alcoholism. Indeed, among women seeking alcohol treatment in this country, "the two phenomena go hand in hand," according to Fillmore.[61] Liver disease also constitutes a more serious threat for women drinkers, and many more have unstable marriages, partners who themselves drink, or families unsympathetic to their treatment. Their self-esteem is lower than drinking men's, their child care responsibilities heavier, their families of origin more chaotic. Many more of them have suffered sexual abuse and tend to turn to the bottle in the face of life crises.[62]

Despite these very particular and pressing feminine needs, however, most of our methods for treating drug and alcohol abuse "were developed by working with men," says Beth Glover Reed, Ph.D., of the University of Michigan School of Social Work.[63] Indeed, it was recovering men in self-help groups, rather than professionals in clinics, who evolved the model that dominates chemical abuse treatment today, the highly successful 12-step programs. Informal, anonymous fellowships of male alcoholics shared and analyzed their mutual problems and gradually built up a body of literature and lore that they found helpful. From this history, Reed believes, arose ideas that reflect masculine rather than feminine realities. Indeed, the very conceptualization of the problem with "its violence, its crime, its drunk driving and work disruption and product disruption by people who are high or drunk on the assembly line," involves "things that happen more often in men."[64]

The key concept of denial, for example, viewed as a major impediment to recovery, "psychodynamically . . . really means the suppression of any kind of negative affect in a very simplified way." Though perhaps prevalent among men, and perhaps reflecting male coping styles, the rejection of one's own feelings of distress does not square with the "very high depression and anxiety scores" seen among chemically dependent women.[65]

Enabling, another key concept from alcohol recovery groups, is "getting picked up by a lot of drug programs and more generic programs" as well, Reed notes. "A mixture of behavioral theory and social systems theory," it denotes practices by the people close to the substance abuser that "enable" the abuse to continue: making excuses for the alcoholic, supplying money, ignoring clues of alcoholism, setting right the intoxication's disastrous consequences, accepting promises that similar catastrophes "won't happen again." Such behavior, Reed suggests, is not inherently alcoholic but rather "gendered. I'm using a women's studies term here on purpose," she explains, "in that much of the way we think about these problems is confounded with male gender role." Progress in recovery can only begin when "enabling" ceases and the addict is forced to face the consequences of the addiction. A woman, it seems, and a wife or mother in particular, is much likelier than a man to "stand by" an addictive family member, doing what she can to hold her home together— a model both of feminine nurturance and loyalty and of classic "enabling."[66] And, indeed, research among HIV-positive users of injection drugs finds that mothers and other female relatives continue to provide material and emotional support. The uninfected female partners of HIV-positive men often even permit their sexual relationships to continue.[67]

WOMEN AND AIDS

To all the damage that drugs and alcohol have done to women's bodies, minds, and spirits over the centuries, the past decade has added a new and yet more terrible danger. Drug addiction, whether a woman's own or her sexual partner's, now serves as a major route of HIV infection. Intravenous drug users can, of course, catch the virus directly from contaminated needles, an ever-present risk among the many addicts who rent "works" in "shooting galleries" or who consider sharing them among friends a sign of trust and solidarity. Because crack cocaine is smoked, it does not expose its users directly to the virus. But the "crack house," where many addicts go both to buy and to use the drug, is generally a scene of uninhibited and anonymous sexuality. In these squalid surroundings, female addicts often trade sex either for money or for the "rocks" themselves.

Worldwide, more than 3 million overwhelmingly young women now have the HIV virus. In large cities in this country and throughout the Americas, Western Europe, and sub-Saharan Africa, more women between 20 and 40 now die of AIDS than of any other cause.[68] Though women still constitute a small proportion of American AIDS cases, their share is rising rapidly, and fastest among African American and Hispanic heterosexual women and injection drug users.[69] Sex has now overtaken the needle as the main vehicle of direct female contagion. Women find themselves in special jeopardy because very few have any means of defense against the virus that is wholly under their own control. Contraceptives that do not impede male pleasure, such as spermicides, sponges, and diaphragms, do not significantly impede HIV either. The one device definitely shown to make sex safer—though not, of course, wholly safe—is the condom, little help to many women. Not only does proper use cut down on many men's enjoyment, it also requires their active cooperation right in the midst of intercourse.

Public health campaigns have concentrated on exhorting people to insist on condoms, but the scanty research that exists on sexual practices among groups at high risk for HIV indicates that use is not generally a strictly individual decision, nor one that women can very often effectively influence. Rather, found IOM's Committee on Substance Abuse and

Mental Health Issues in AIDS Research, consistent condom use is "a characteristic of social relationships rather than an individual attribute." People sometimes used them and sometimes did not, one Brooklyn study showed, depending on whom they were with, how they felt, or any one of a number of unknown factors.[70]

In general, only about two-thirds of drug injectors infected with HIV consistently used condoms during sex with non-drug users.[71] Condom use in the general population is probably a good deal lower even than that sorry figure. Fewer than one-fifth of those with multiple partners, and about 10% of those whose partners are known to be risky, use condoms every time.[72] Adding to the danger of unprotected sex are the other venereal diseases and infections that help speed the virus's passage from person to person. Widespread where condom use is scarce, syphillis, gonorrhea, herpes, and genital warts all increase a person's likelihood of picking up the infection during vaginal or oral sex, as do the burns and sores that often afflict the mouths and lips of crack smokers.[73]

Americans simply do not seem to have generally adopted the condom habit. Indeed, the AIDS committee observes, "Many of those at risk for HIV infections—whether through sex or drug use—do not recognize the danger they face." What's more, "even when they do, knowledge alone is not enough to effect behavior change to reduce their risks."[74]

In the poor minority communities where HIV is spreading most rapidly, knowledge may be essentially irrelevant to a woman's fate. The theoretical models that have shaped our national approach to AIDS education assume, in the committee's words, "that individuals are acting in an intentional and volitional manner" when having sex; that, in other words, they voluntarily and knowingly choose to take part and have some control over their actions.[75] Clearly, for large numbers of women, this assumption drastically distorts reality. We saw in the last chapter how even well-educated girls come to sexuality poorly equipped to influence male decisions; how much worse is the bargaining power of poor, badly educated ones! And in the life-and-death negotiations surrounding exposure to HIV, various subgroup customs severely increase women's already dangerous disadvantage.

In certain cultures, Scrimshaw reports, including some prominent in the United States, a woman does not "have a choice on sex when [she's] tired" or at any other time she does not wish to satisfy her man's desire. Some Latin American women, she continues, use the expression " 'Abuso del hombre,' which means 'abuse by the man,' [as a] euphemism for sex. Or, 'me uso anoche' [which means] 'he used me last night,' is a euphemism for saying 'we had sex last night.' "[76] Women's " 'permanent inequality' in status and power" separates many of them from their men and undermines their freedom of action, the AIDS committee observes.[77]

When sex is a masculine prerogative, tradition generally also dictates that "women should not initiate discussion of sexual practices or try to change their male partner's sexual behavior," the AIDS committee goes on. A man may well see a request that he use a condom "as an act of distrust and suspicion, rather than an act of caring, respect and mutuality" as portrayed in the public health campaigns.[78] What's more, "violence and abuse are a daily reality in the lives of many addicted women and among women with male partners who are addicted." Recent research even "suggests that fear of the partner's anger" should the subject of protection arise strongly influences "condom use among Hispanic/Latina women." In a stunning understatement, the committee concludes that to stem the spread of AIDS, "programs that highlight the importance of open communication between women and their partners . . . may be of limited value."[79]

If culture does not allow women to defend their health, then technology—in the form of some protective barrier that women can control and men will accept—may be the only hope. A "female condom" marketed under the name "Reality" came on the U.S. market in January 1994. Composed of a plastic sheath held in the vaginal canal by a pair of plastic rings, it combines features of the diaphragm and the condom and overcomes several of the important objections to the familiar male device. The woman can insert it before intercourse, rather than having to interrupt lovemaking. Lying loosely inside the vagina, it interferes less with male sensation, breaks less often, and covers a greater portion of the female tissue exposed to STD infection. Nor need it be removed immediately after ejaculation. Indeed, limited testing shows that both women and men, including commercial sex workers and their clients, find it more acceptable and feasible than the alternative device. Despite these "promising results," however, the AIDS committee notes that research has not yet definitively proven Reality's effectiveness as either a contraceptive or a barrier against infection, nor is it yet widely available in the United States.[80]

Nor, of course, does such a device offer any relief to the many women, mostly Hispanic and African American, already infected, nor to the children they continue to bear. For many poor women, the AIDS committee believes, "the role of mother is the primary pathway to greater social status and respect in their communities. Particularly for those women devalued" by their status as drug users, motherhood "takes on added importance." A woman "torn between the value placed on children and motherhood and the possibility that the child may be born HIV positive" has little chance of succeeding at contraception.[81]

Then, when her own infection erupts into full-blown AIDS, she finds herself both "consumed with worry" over the care of her children after her impending death and "less likely to have the support of a mate" than women without HIV. Should the children also have the virus, their often desperately ill mother has the additional concern that they "may suffer even greater discrimination" in the already overburdened foster care system. With a support network "more constricted than that of other AIDS patients," this hapless soul must also contend with poverty that keeps her from both "obtaining the expensive drugs needed to treat AIDS" and "traveling long distances for the limited amount of care that may be available."[82]

For women, then, HIV and AIDS present dangers, issues, challenges, and needs quite unlike those facing men. Scientific assumptions based on masculine circumstances—that an individual can control the terms of sexual contact, that the possibility exists of protecting oneself, that a support system will step in to provide care during illness—are jeopardizing the health of countless women and their children. Only through a drastic rethinking of our approach to the disease and its spread can we hope to alleviate vast future female suffering.

MOVING ON

As American women move into their forties, the great majority have completed their families. They have also, often unwittingly, made decisions that will affect their health for many years ahead, just as decisions made in childhood and adolescence have already helped shape their adult lives. The timing of a woman's children, for example, influences her risk of breast cancer, which starts to rise slowly in the fifth decade and then more rapidly in the decades beyond.

For all its sociological drawbacks, childbearing before 20 does bring at least one advantage, albeit a benefit that hardly outweighs the costs in lost opportunities. It markedly reduces breast cancer risk. Waiting until 30 to give birth, an increasingly common choice among the educated, on the other hand, raises this risk, as does having no children at all. One's choice of contraception can also affect future chances of disease. The Pill and other hormonal types protect against ovarian cancer. Barrier types like the diaphragm and the condom cut down on sexually transmitted diseases. Having had many lovers has the opposite effect and also raises the risk of cervical cancer.

A woman who has been physically active, kept her weight under control, and eaten sensibly has also cut her risks of osteoporosis, heart disease, and reproductive cancers. Whatever health choices a woman made in the early stages of her life, as she moves into middle age, she will soon begin to see the rewards or errors of her ways.

NOTES

1. *Science and Babies: Private Decisions, Public Dilemmas*, 1-2.
2. *Developing New Contraceptives: Obstacles and Opportunities*, 14.
3. Ibid.
4. Ibid., 20.
5. Ibid., 20-1.
6. Ibid., 19-20.
7. Ibid., 13.
8. Ibid., 26-7.
9. Ibid., 22.
10. Ibid.
11. Ibid., 22-3.
12. *Science and Babies*, 44.
13. IOM 1992 Annual Meeting, 139.
14. *Developing New Contraceptives*, 28.
15. Ibid., 30.
16. *Science and Babies*, 60.
17. Ibid., 57.
18. IOM 1992 Annual Meeting, 137.
19. *Science and Babies*, 7.
20. Ibid., 53.

21. *Clinical Applications of Mifespristone (RU 486) and Other Antiprogestins: Assessing the Science and Recommending a Research Agenda*, 72.

22. Ibid.

23. Ibid., 92.

24. Ibid., 72.

25. Ibid., 92.

26. Ibid., 93.

27. Ibid., 6.

28. Ibid., 3.

29. *Science and Babies*, 15.

30. Ibid., 19.

31. Ibid., 15.

32. Ibid., 5.

33. Ibid., 18.

34. Ibid., 21.

35. Ibid., 21-3, passim.

36. Ibid., 36.

37. Ibid., 98.

38. Ibid., 97.

39. Ibid., 96.

40. Ibid., 98.

41. Ibid., 107.

42. Ibid., 97.

43. Ibid., 105.

44. *Medical Professional Liability and the Delivery of Obstetrical Care*, Vol. II, 34.

45. *Healthy People 2000: Citizens Chart the Course*, 171.

46. *Access to Health Care in America*, 52.

47. *Medical Professional Liability*, Vol. I, 26.

48. *Science and Babies*, 107.

49. *Nutrition During Pregnancy*, 51.

50. *Medical Professional Liability*, Vol. II, 28-30, passim.

51. Ibid., 30.

52. Ibid., 28.

53. Ibid., 32.

54. Ibid., 34-5.

55. *Reducing Risks for Mental Disorders: Frontiers for Preventive Intervention Research*, 65.

56. Assessing Future Research Needs: Mental and Addictive Disorders in Women (Transcript), 184.

57. *Health and Behavior, Frontiers of Research in the Biobehavioral Sciences*, 165.

58. Assessing Future Research Needs (Transcript), 129.

59. Ibid., 130.

60. *Broadening the Base of Treatment for Alcohol Problems*, 356-7.

61. Assessing Future Research Needs (Transcript), 131.

62. *Broadening the Base of Treatment for Alcohol Problems*, 357.

63. Assessing Future Research Needs (Transcript), 243.

64. Ibid., 243-5.

65. Ibid., 244.

66. Ibid., 242-3.

67. *AIDS and Behavior: An Integrated Approach*, 91.

68. Ibid., 112.

69. Ibid., 95.

70. Ibid., 75.
71. Ibid.
72. Ibid., 83.
73. Ibid., 50.
74. Ibid., 83.
75. Ibid., 7.
76. Scrimshaw (1991), 24.
77. *AIDS and Behavior*, 96.
78. Ibid., 92-3.
79. Ibid., 96-7.
80. Ibid., 112-3.
81. Ibid., 97.
82. Ibid.

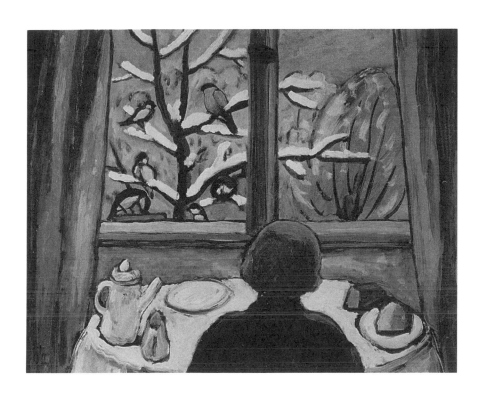

Gabriele Munter
Breakfast of the Birds (1934)
Oil on board
The National Museum of Women in the Arts
Gift of Wallace and Wilhelmina Holladay

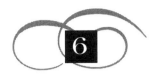

Health Through the
Life Span:
Menopause and Beyond

At some point several decades after she began to menstruate—
usually sometime during her late forties or early fifties—a
woman's monthly periods cease. Certain women, especially
smokers, pass this milestone on the early side, in the early to mid-forties or
even before; others pass it later than average. Cessation before the age of
40 is technically considered "premature," a diagnosis that in itself does not
imply abnormality but sometimes indicates conditions that need treatment.

Over a period of time, on a schedule largely determined by
genetics, a woman's aging ovaries stop responding to the hormonal signal
that has, since early in her second decade, regularly urged them to send
forth an egg. Her cycles may shorten or become erratic. Her flow becomes increasingly scant. She ovulates less and less often. Whether gradually over a year or two or abruptly in a matter of months, she experiences
the menopause, the point at which her menstrual cycles and her reproductive opportunities permanently end (unless, of course, she chooses to
try for a geriatric pregnancy through the high-tech treatments that have
recently made worldwide headlines).

For some women, menopause comes as a sudden side effect of
medical intervention, such as radiation or hormone treatments for cancer
or surgical removal of the uterus and ovaries. However it happens, though,

a woman crosses a significant divide into an era with its own distinct health risks.

A vast and not very flattering folklore details the supposed vagaries of "the change of life"—wild and unpredictable mood swings, debilitating hot flashes, snappishness, crying jags, headaches, loss of libido. Most women, however, pass through the climacteric, as this transitional phase is technically known, without undue discomfort or distress. Some notice no symptoms at all. Others suffer extreme effects. On average, though, American women find this a period of at most moderate and certainly manageable annoyance. When a year has passed since her last menses, a woman has technically reached her menopause.

This marks her arrival at the third—though usually the second longest—major portion of her biological life. The average American woman now lives up to three decades after her menopause—more than twice as long as the period leading up to her puberty. The increasing numbers of women now continuing on into their nineties and beyond can easily spend as many or even more years in the post-reproductive state as they did in the supposedly "central" reproductive stage of life. Given the great and rapidly changing significance of both this life stage and the complex and highly variable physiological processes that usher it in, medical science knows remarkably little about the issues, risks, and opportunities that women face during and after menopause. As we have seen, both medical science and the society that supports it have until very recently considered menopause the end of a woman's "useful" life and the years that follow it a sort of physiological caboose containing not much of interest except tedium, depression, and decline.

Though considerable attention has gone to the diseases that afflict and kill large numbers of older men, their manifestations in women traditionally got a good deal less, in part because women—at least since the great medical advances in this century's early decades—just "naturally" live longer. For the centuries before those great steps forward, relatively few women—or men, for that matter—lived beyond or even until the age of menopause, and those who did were exceptionally hardy and fortunate specimens. More pressing concerns like rampant infectious disease, heart disease, and cancer had a greater call on researchers' time. Only within the past decade or so have issues like osteoporosis and breast cancer, major concerns of women's sixth decade and beyond, begun to demand a larger share of resources.

IMAGES OF AGING

In the United States, many women fear that menopause signals the end of their important womanly roles. In traditional societies around the world, though, its arrival heralds, for socially well-situated people, unprecedented and often eagerly awaited opportunities. To paraphrase Abraham Lincoln, the end of childbearing represents a literal and usually very welcome "new birth of freedom." Age in this context means not a decline in personal worth but the attainment of "autonomy and independence" as one finally reaches "the matriarch stage," Scrimshaw says. Any one who has "read the wonderful novel, *One Hundred Years of Solitude*," she adds, "will think of Ursula, . . . the archetype of this matriarch. And matriarchs actually have a lot of power and a lot of independence. And if you want to skip over a few continents to India and think of the power of the mother-in-law, the power of the senior women in the household or the power of the senior women in Africa, you'll see that there's more autonomy."[1]

Indeed, in societies around the world, whether in peasant Europe, the Muslim Middle East, or Pearl Buck's China, female adulthood has traditionally been a trek from the utter powerlessness of a young woman valued essentially for her ability to produce offspring but feared for her ability to dishonor the family name, toward the prestige and relative comfort of the female head of the household and often, should her husband predecease her, the unrivaled domestic ruler. In those societies where property descends in the female line, the matriarch also exercises authority as an economic and often a political actor. In many traditional cultures, as, for example, among certain African, Creole, and Native American peoples, older women also play important religious, spiritual, and medical roles as elders, wise women, diviners, healers, and teachers.

Past the possibility of pregnancy, a woman no longer need fear the unexpected and possibly unwanted arrival of additional hungry mouths. Beyond that, having gradually lost her sexual desirability and then definitively lost her ability to demonstrate her mate's sexual prowess with a new pregnancy, she frees herself of the constraints, tensions, and pressures that male honor or jealousy imposed on her during her years as a valuable sex object. Far from any longer needing a chaperone, she now becomes one. Far from figuring as a pawn in her elders' matrimonial strategies, she now takes part as a major player in the wheeling and dealing. Far from being an ignored nobody in the councils of the powerful, she now exercises a forceful voice in family and even community affairs. Far from enduring backbreaking work while pregnant or nursing, she now supervises younger women, her daughters or daughters-in-law, who do much of the household's labor.

Assuming that a woman had a sufficient number of children of the proper genders, and that she belongs to family of adequate social and economic standing within her community, and that her household hews to the traditional norms, the end of her fertility in certain respects promises one of the most rewarding periods of her life. Of course, not all women in traditional societies get to enjoy this crowning stage. "This autonomy and independence comes after a lot of the reproductive risk and after a lot of the growth risk," Scrimshaw cautions, risks that huge numbers of women bearing children in deprived circumstances or suffering chronic diseases without adequate medical care, simply do not survive. For Scrimshaw's "missing women," "in other words, it comes too late."[2]

Even if large numbers in traditional societies miss out on enjoying this culminating life stage, however, it still stands in stark contrast to the treatment that older American women have come to expect. In a society composed of small, mobile nuclear families rather than of large, stationary extended households, older women lose rather than gain prestige and importance as their children mature into parenthood. Instead of becoming heads of an expanding concern, they become members of one- or two-person households. Instead of moving to a position honored for its power, many face demotion as they lose their physical appeal, often the basis for ties to men in a society that bases marriage on love. Instead of achieving relative material comfort, many find themselves displaced by divorce or widowhood.

Our society has for generations depicted postmenopausal women as insignificant and not very attractive: "blue-haired" ladies in "tennis shoes," baleful mothers-in-law, dried-up old hags. Even the ancient pagan wise woman has been transformed into the cackling witch. Now and then a lovable old granny appears on the scene bearing a platter of oatmeal cookies or beaming down a spanking white Thanksgiving table or dispensing family lore to a pampered grandchild. In general, though, whether as Jiggs's Maggie or Edith Bunker or one of the "Golden Girls" in their shared Florida rambler, the woman past childbearing has not been a figure of gravity or substance in American culture.

How much and how quickly the recent revolution in women's roles will affect this image—and older women's images of themselves— still remains to be seen. But now that "postmenopausal" describes Supreme Court justices, university presidents, corporate executives, prominent surgeons, Nobel laureates, army generals, and even, in a few cases, movie stars, and now that less celebrated women have come to realize that the years after their children are grown represent an opportunity for largely unfettered attainment, we may witness the transformation of this third stage of female life.

GETTING THE FACTS

If they are not yet considered glamorous, though, the years after menopause at least are beginning to garner increased scientific and media attention. Over the past decade or two, women have begun to demand more information about their concerns. Not until the early 1990s, though, did the National Institutes of Health, under the prodding of its first female director, Bernadine Healey, M.D., undertake to do a comprehensive study of several of the major health issues after menopause. The Women's Health Initiative (WHI), projected to cost $625 million over 15 years and to involve 160,000 postmenopausal women at 45 clinical centers and additional thousands in community-based studies, officially got under way in 1993.[3]

The largest project ever funded in NIH history, WHI will investigate ways of preventing three major killers, cardiovascular disease, breast cancer, and osteoporosis.[4] These diseases arise after menopause because the most visible sign of the changes taking place in a woman's body, the cessation of her periods, is really only a symptom of much deeper and more important events. In a process every bit as profound in its physical (and often, its social) ramifications as puberty, a woman's entire hormonal balance once again shifts. Her supply of the natural estrogen produced by the ovaries drops sharply, and the many tissues throughout the body affected by that hormone begin to undergo change. Among other things, the bones and vaginal lining thin, the blood cholesterol level rises, the heart and circulatory system begin to deteriorate, the skin more rapidly wrinkles. Rates of heart disease and osteoporosis, the extremely painful and dangerous disease that embrittles the bones, begin to rise. Sexual intercourse may become uncomfortable or even painful.

To forestall these problems—especially the life-threatening decay of bones, heart, and blood vessels—many experts now recommend that women replace their lost natural estrogen with therapeutic doses of the hormone. Taken alone, however, this so-called "unopposed estrogen" is known to encourage cancer of the endometrium, or uterine lining. Women who retain a uterus are thus also advised to take doses of progestins, hormones of pregnancy, which lower this risk.

Beyond these effects, however, not enough is known about the consequences of long-term hormone replacement therapy (HRT) on overall survival; to find out is one of WHI's major goals. Specifically, the study will explore how much HRT actually lessens the incidence of osteoporosis and cardiovascular disease and whether, as some suspect, it also increases the risk of breast cancer. In addition, it will examine the effect of low-fat diets on breast cancer and heart disease.

Women badly need these questions answered. Although many now take HRT to counter unpleasant symptoms of the climacteric, especially hot flashes, these are usually transitory and the therapy often ceases in a matter of months. Only about 5% of women now continue hormones over a period of years, which researchers believe is necessary to gain the potentially lifesaving benefits. Uncertainty about the long term often makes both women and their doctors hesitate to continue with a powerful prescription drug for years on a strictly preventative basis.

The cardiovascular benefits of estrogen replacement are clear, as is the reduction in hip and other bone fractures in white women. But does the addition of progestin negate these advantages? Do these hormones increase the possibility of breast cancer? If so, do the benefits of

HRT outweigh the risks for women who are not at high risk for tumors? The answers to these questions, alas, are at least a decade away.[5]

One thing is clear, however: in this third part of life, health choices made often unwittingly years, even decades, earlier, come definitively home to roost. The incidence of breast and other reproductive cancers begins to rise steeply, reflecting, at least in part, women's reproductive, contraceptive, and sexual histories. Regular cancer screening, through mammograms and Pap smears, now becomes especially important, particularly since evidence suggests that these tests may well have more predictive power in older than in younger women. Nor has any statistician found an age at which these screenings can be safely stopped.[6] Three decades or so after adolescence, smoking also begins to take its own toll in cancers, strokes, heart conditions, and lung disease. Bone loss accelerates, especially among those who smoke or who do not exercise.

Inactivity, always more common among women than men, increases as people get older. More and more individuals meet the definition of sedentary by failing to exercise at least three times a week or at least 20 minutes a session. Age, however, in itself cannot account for the accelerating drop in physical powers that many sedentary people experience. Fully "50 percent of the decline frequently attributed to physiological aging is, in reality, disuse atrophy resulting from inactivity in an industrial world," notes IOM's Committee on Health Promotion and Disability Prevention for the Second Fifty Years.[7] The belief that they were "too delicate" for sports in their younger years now truly helps make women frail as they approach their older ones. And the same technologies that have freed American women from untold household drudgery, that made childbirth safe, and that produced the cures for many diseases have allowed many individuals to put themselves at risk for needless physical deterioration.

AGING AS A FEMALE ISSUE

But if the inevitability of universal rapid decline is a myth, another common perception about aging is not: the large and growing preponderance of women among America's older citizens. Our mammalian relatives do not show any substantial female advantage in longevity,

nor, in fact, did our foremothers and forefathers at the turn of the twentieth century. Since then, however, the difference between American men's
and women's life expectancy has markedly widened. Death in childbirth
has gone from an ever-present danger to a freak accident. Lifestyle factors,
probably prominent among them the formerly much lower female use of
tobacco, probably play a major part in the difference. With cigarette smoking now widespread among young women, however, and with lung cancer, one of the disease's most deadly and least treatable forms, now the
leading cancer killer among women, females may begin losing ground.

For the time being, though, and for the immediately foresee-
able future, women form a larger percentage of their age group the older
they get. At age 65 they number 1.5 females for every male, by age 85,
2.5:1.[8] The average wife can expect to outlive her husband by nearly a
decade.[9] For women, therefore, widowhood is an extremely common
feature of old age. Two-thirds of the women over 75, but less than one-
quarter of the men, are widowed.[10] This imbalance produces, among
other things, the scene "in nursing homes of the one man with a bevy of
women hovering over him, often to his dismay," Cohler says.[11] It also
produces a real demographic bar to finding a new mate. More than half of
the men widowed by age 55 marry, but many fewer of the women. In the
later decades of life, in fact, women marry at the rate of men two decades
their senior.[12]

FACING LOSS

Losing a husband has two major consequences that bear importantly on women's health: the stress of the bereavement itself and the
tendency that widowhood produces to live alone. "Only those who themselves die young escape the pain of losing someone they love through
death," observes IOM's Committee for the Study of Health Consequences
of the Stress of Bereavement. Whenever researchers have studied the
health of bereaved persons, "what they learned lent scientific credence to
what poets, novelists and playwrights had long suggested. Bereavement
affects people in different ways, and for some, especially those whose
health is already compromised, bereavement can exacerbate mental and
physical health problems and even lead to death."[13]

In many ways the manifestations of grief resemble those of depression. Both involve profound sadness, anxiety, and agitation. Both entail sleeplessness, loss of appetite and interests, intense emotional distress. But grief, unlike depression, is not a disease, and neither society nor the grieving person herself considers it as such. Rather, every culture provides mourning customs that channel feelings and demarcate a period for the normal and expected reaction to great loss. Every culture accords the bereaved a special status and time to abandon the normal responsibilities incompatible with their sorrow. Every culture affords its members a means of expressing respect and condolence to the bereft family. Indeed, the person who does not grieve at the appropriate time is the one considered disordered.

In its sheer normality, therefore, "bereavement may be compared to pregnancy," the committee suggests. "Both are naturally occurring conditions for which many individuals seek medical attention." The grieving "may be prescribed tranquilizers, sleeping pills and sedatives, but they seldom seek psychiatric care." Nor do they normally feel the utter hopelessness and often suicidal despair of the clinically depressed. In a classic insight, Freud "contended that most people in the grieving state feel there has been a loss or emptiness in the world around them, while depressed patients feel empty within. A pervasive loss of self-regard or self-esteem is common in depressed patients but not in most grieving individuals," the committee adds.[14]

Surprisingly enough, despite older people's intimate acquaintance with grief through the accumulating losses of parents, spouses, siblings, friends, sometimes even children, the disease of depression actually afflicts them less than it does their juniors. The highest rates of depression found among elderly persons without medical problems are lower than those found among the young. Depressed older persons tend to live in nursing homes and, especially, to suffer dementia.[15] "There is a stereotype that older adults experience lower morale as contrasted with their younger counterparts," Cohler notes, as well as "greater psychiatric impairment." In fact, however, studies show that three-quarters of those surveyed "report their morale to be good to excellent, with only a small minority reporting a memory problem . . . or increased loneliness," he continues.[16] "Older adults are not by and large lonely," Cohler goes on. "What we do know is that older adults . . . and particularly older women, tend to prefer reminiscence about the past to actual social participation." He tells of a woman living in a nursing home whose hours sitting alone at a card table laying out bridge hands had convinced staff members that she was depressed. "It turned out that she was reliving her lifetime in which she and her husband and their best friends played bridge together," remembrances that made it possible for her to face her present life.[17]

A widow's passage has been described as going from "being a wife to being a widow to being a woman."[18] No longer half of a couple, she faces the challenge of becoming a whole person in her own right. Indeed, the more dependent on others a widow remains after her loss, the worse her adjustment to her new circumstances tends to be. If she lacks some of the "survival" skills of independent living—if she needs others to drive her around, for example, or do her banking or pay her bills—she is likelier to be anxious, isolated, and depressed than a woman in charge of her own affairs.[19]

FROM OWN HOME TO NURSING HOME

Losing her husband deprives a woman not only of her role as a wife, but also of her domestic partner. For that reason, women constitute four-fifths of all elderly persons who live alone. At every age, at least twice as many older women as older men live alone.[20] In addition to facing much worse odds than men in finding a new spouse, women generally "could not engage in new relationships soon after their husbands' deaths without feeling disloyal," reports the bereavement committee. "In contrast, widowers did not seem to feel that a new relationship would conflict with their commitment to their deceased spouses. In fact, widowers who established a new quasi-marital relationship a few months after bereavement expected their new partners to be sympathetic to their continued grieving."[21]

Sentiment and demography therefore combine to render three-quarters of women between 65 and 74 and four-fifths of those older than 75 the solitary inhabitants of their own households.[22] The lack of someone else at home can become crucial as women pass from being "young-old, roughly 65 to 75," in Cohler's words, to being "old-old, 75 plus."

Most in the first category remain unencumbered by handicapping conditions. Most in the second "report some sorts of chronic disability," he goes on, "although what a physician reports as a disability may not be what a person himself reports." He tells of a woman with "both cancer and heart disease, and she says, 'Yes, but you ought to see my neighbor.' " Health, he concludes, is "very much a subjective experience, not as rated by a physician."[23]

Eventually, though, as disabilities increase, the objective inability to care for oneself often overwhelms the most optimistic subjective reality. A woman living alone is less likely than one living with a spouse to have someone who can care for her at home during infirmity. Indeed, the major determinant of who moves into a nursing home proves not to be how sick the person is but how available care is at home.[21] Widowed parents often receive a great deal of help from grown children, sometimes moving into their homes for that purpose. In long-term and degenerative chronic diseases, though, the strain of adding an ailing elder often proves too great for the family to bear. For an individual who cannot maintain an independent household, a nursing home or other institution may well be the only feasible solution.

LOOKING AHEAD

The picture painted here of health in the later years depicts the present generation of older women. The "baby boomer" generation now approaching and passing through menopause, however, may retouch the composition, as they have altered the contours of every other life stage they have passed through. And the generations younger still may well totally rearrange some important aspects of many American women's portraits. Beginning menstruation at younger and younger ages, smoking in larger and larger numbers, marrying later or not at all, giving birth either very early or very late, divorcing often, working for pay most of their adult lives, juggling multiple—and often conflicting—roles during the reproductive years, attaining unprecedented self-sufficiency through their own earnings, they may make many elements of our current picture obsolete.

Whatever the future holds, though, and however much women's biographies may diverge from their mothers' and in important respects come to resemble men's, one paramount principle will remain. A woman's health status will always reflect the choices she made from among the array available in her time and place. The answer to Scrimshaw's question "Why women?" will always be found in the concrete circumstances in which individual women pass the days and years of their lives.

NOTES

1. Scrimshaw (1991), 8.
2. Ibid.
3. *An Assessment of the NIH Women's Health Initiative*, 1.
4. Ibid.
5. *The Second Fifty Years: Promoting Health and Preventing Disability*, 88-9.
6. Ibid., 141-3.
7. Ibid., 225.
8. *Medicare: A Strategy for Quality Assurance*, Vol. I, 71.
9. Assessing Future Research Needs: Mental and Addictive Disorders in Women (Transcript), 167.
10. Ibid., 165.
11. Ibid.
12. *Bereavement: Reactions, Consequences, and Care*, 24.
13. Ibid., 3-4.
14. Ibid., 19.
15. *The Second Fifty Years*, 203-4.
16. Assessing Future Research Needs (Transcript), 168.
17. Ibid.
18. N. Golan, *Social Work*, v. 20, quoted in *Bereavement*, 74.
19. *Bereavement*, 61.
20. *Medicare*, Vol. I, 74.
21. *Bereavement*, 75.
22. *Medicare*, Vol. I, 74.
23. Assessing Future Research Needs (Transcript), 164.
24. *Allied Health Services: Avoiding Crises*, 261.

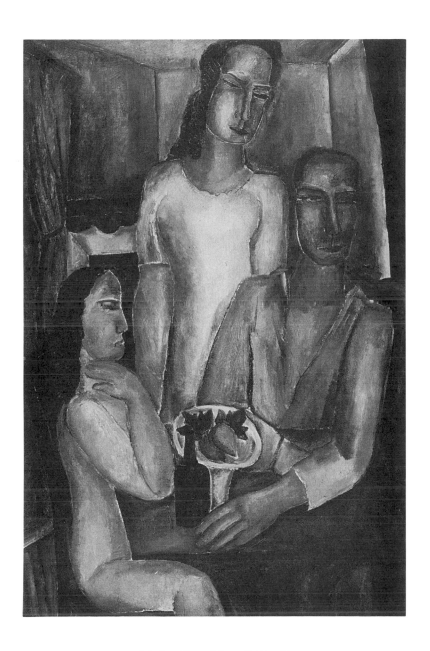

Valentine Henriette Prax
The Family (n.d.)
Oil on canvas
The National Museum of Women in the Arts
Gift of Mrs. Philip D. Wiedel

Eating for a Healthy Life

Many women spend significant portions of their lives thinking about food. From the moment that a preadolescent gets the first inkling of the changes happening to her body to the day an octogenarian gives away the pots and dishes she will not be needing at the retirement home, a substantial portion of nearly every day goes into considering what should or should not be on her own and other people's plates. So central is this concern that, according to survivors' accounts, women (and men) starving in World War II concentration camps passed the time by discussing menus and recipes for the feasts they planned to prepare after their liberation.

But in a lifetime spent concentrating on cooking and eating; in decade upon decade of perusing articles and clipping recipes from magazines and newspapers, of seeking nutritional counsel from obstetricians and pediatricians, of studying labels and assessing produce in supermarkets, of fretting about unwanted pounds, of helping a mate cut back on fat or salt or caffeine, of sharing kitchen tips with friends, and, often, of putting three squares (or at least one or two) on the table nearly every day of the year, many an American woman neglects to find out how best to eat for her own health.

Despite the most stable and abundant larder in human history, despite grocery prices far cheaper as a proportion of income than in many other countries, despite food choices from abalone to zucchini, American girls and women typically eat diets that put them at risk for certain health problems. And these nutrition-related conditions differ somewhat from those most common in men.

So striking a pattern of behavior is not, of course, an accident.

First, and most obviously, women's bodies face nutritional challenges that men's never do. The monthly menstrual flow taxes their stores of iron. Pregnancy and lactation place immense burdens on both women's bodies and their ability to consume the nutrients they need to create and nourish a new life without depleting the nutritional stores they need to maintain their own health. Then, after menopause, due to the drop in estrogens and the protection they impart, a variety of chronic diseases apparently related at least in part to diet choices made during earlier decades arise: osteoporosis, cardiovascular disorders, and reproductive cancers.

Despite growing evidence for a diet-disease connection, however, such ties have been difficult to nail down definitively. Specific mechanisms of action often remain elusive. International comparisons, for example, clearly show a relationship between a nation's breast cancer rate and the level of fat in its people's diet, but science has yet to isolate the precise biological elements of this connection.

In nutritional epidemiology, the science that studies the interplay of food and illness, "new hypotheses are easily generated because so many diet variables allow many comparisons to be made," warns Elizabeth Barrett-Connor, M.D., professor of epidemiology at the University of California, San Diego, School of Medicine. Conflicting studies have suggested, for example, that eating yogurt both does and does not raise the risk of ovarian cancer. Further investigations have shown an even more complicated apparent connection between cancer risk, use of birth control pills—which seem to provide some protection against malignancy of the ovaries—and consumption of dairy products.

Such a "rather convoluted association is biologically plausible," Barrett-Connor notes. A diet high in the milk sugar lactose results in a high intake of the sugar galactose, which in turn stimulates production of gonadotrophins, hormones lowered by the Pill. This theory serves to "highlight another characteristic of epidemiological studies of diet and disease: it is possible to find and explain almost anything," she goes on. "The metabolic pathways of humans are sufficiently complicated, as are our other behaviors (e.g., taking oral contraceptives), that we can explain almost any nutrition-disease association we find." The lesson Barrett-Connor draws: researchers must guard against becoming "prematurely enamored with causality." That's why, she says, a large, well-controlled trial like the Women's Health Initiative (WHI) will play an important role in distinguishing "which associations are causal and which are coincidental."[1]

Other methodological problems lie in wait for the researcher stalking connections between diet and disease. "Social mores may conceal the truth about diet," Barrett-Connor goes on. "Hampering scientists' efforts to track fat, for example, is the fact that "it is no longer socially acceptable in California to admit to anyone that you eat three eggs for breakfast, consume red meat twice a day, never cut the fat off anything." When "the lay media constantly remind us of how we should eat and drink," people may give interviewers fashionable rather than truthful answers. And, "if women are more educated about good food habits than men, and I expect they are, then their reported diet could more readily obscure diet-disease associations" simply because they keep up on current thinking about what's sensible and what's not.[2] As yet, therefore, only a few specific ills have been traced to particular eating habits.

In large part because of these difficulties, experts emphasize that good nutrition does not depend on certain specific edibles that act as "magic bullets" against particular problems, like oat bran or fish oil, to name two that became national fads. Nor does it lie in specific vitamins or minerals gulped down in supplements. Rather, it entails a judicious selection of ordinary foods, which should be the "normal vehicle for delivering nutrients," according to Janet King, Ph.D., professor of nutritional sciences at the University of California, Berkeley.[3] Only in special circumstances should a healthy woman require dietary supplements, and those should be carefully tailored to her particular needs. Otherwise, the neighborhood grocery can provide virtually all the nourishment necessary for health.

To face the special challenges of female life, and to reduce their risk of chronic disease, experts advise American women to follow the same general guidelines that ought to mold everyone's menu. IOM's Committee on Diet and Health has formulated nine simple instructions that make it easy, in the committee's words, to "eat for life" (see Table 7-1). A book by that name, published by the National Academy Press in 1992, gives complete details.

The committee believes that a varied diet low in fat; high in grains, vegetables, and fruits; and moderate in protein, salt, and sweets will provide the building blocks of health for every age beyond infancy and very early childhood. To cut the excessive fat typical of American meals, the ancient concept of "our daily bread" ought once again to form the foundation of our food choices, with complex carbohydrates like pastas, cereals, and whole grain breads accounting for our largest single food category. We should also "strive for five" servings of vegetables and fruits daily, as the supermarket slogan goes, emphasizing the citrus family, yellows, oranges and greens. Low-fat meat, fish, poultry, or legume dishes should appear in small portions two or three times each day to provide protein.

Women in particular also need two or three servings of high-calcium, and preferably low-fat, milk products daily. Sweets, sugars, and oils ought to show up sparingly at best. These high-calorie foods provide few nutrients and can crowd out other, more nourishing possibilities. The same goes for alcohol. Given these choices, American women who are not pregnant or nursing or who do not have other specific health problems ought to attain adequate nourishment without resorting to supplements.

A LOSING PROPOSITION

Good food habits should start early in life, because, as we have seen, they quite literally build the framework for future health. But a nefarious combination of physiological demands and social influences conspires to rob many American girls of, among other things, their best shot at what Barrett-Connor calls "the optimal bone mass to which they are genetically entitled," adding to their risk of osteoporosis and fracture in their later years.[4] During the very years that they need to be laying down the calcium supply in bone that must last a lifetime, as well as other

TABLE 7-1 The Nine Dietary Guidelines

1. Reduce total fat intake to 30 percent or less of your total calorie consumption. Reduce saturated fatty acid intake to less than 10 percent of calories. Reduce cholesterol intake to less than 300 milligrams daily.

2. Eat five or more servings of a combination of vegetables and fruits daily, especially green and yellow vegetables and citrus fruits. Also, increase your intake of starches and other complex carbohydrates by eating six or more daily servings of a combination of breads, cereals, and legumes.

3. Eat a reasonable amount of protein, maintaining your protein consumption at moderate levels.

4. Balance the amount of food you eat with the amount of exercise you get to maintain appropriate body weight.

5. It is not recommended that you drink alcohol. If you do drink alcoholic beverages, limit the amount you drink in a single day to no more than two cans of beer, two small glasses of wine, or two average cocktails. Pregnant women should avoid alcoholic beverages.

6. Limit the amount of salt (sodium chloride) that you eat to 6 grams (slightly more than 1 teaspoon of salt) per day or less. Limit the use of salt in cooking and avoid adding it to food at the table. Salty foods, including highly processed salty foods, salt-preserved foods, and salt-pickled foods, should be eaten sparingly, if at all.

7. Maintain adequate calcium intake.

8. Avoid taking dietary supplements in excess of the U.S. Recommended Daily Allowances in any one day.

9. Maintain an optimal level of fluoride in your diet and particularly in the diets of your children when their baby and adult teeth are forming.

SOURCE: Institute of Medicine, *Eat for Life: The Food and Nutrition Board's Guide to Reducing Your Risk of Chronic Disease*, 1992, page 6.

nutritional stores to see them through the challenges ahead, they decrease their intake of dairy products as they face an intense and growing cultural pressure that competes with their need for a nutritious, well-balanced diet.

Women around the world, of course, face social challenges to eating properly. In many developing countries, Scrimshaw notes, food is scarce for everyone, but social practices make the situation even worse for women. They frequently eat only after the men and boys have finished, for example, getting only what is left over, rarely the most desirable foods. The best, most nutritious delicacies may in fact be specifically earmarked for males.

"Both in absolute terms and in relation to recommended daily allowance[s], women and girls eat less than men and boys," Scrimshaw says. "Deficiency, of course, is greatest among the lowest socioeconomic class. And women get less food because they're seen as both less needy and also less deserving. The physical size and strength of men is equated with greater needs, to a degree where women [in developing countries] don't get enough."[5]

Even nutritional experts may reinforce this misconception, she notes. A health program in Guatemala, for example, proposed giving male plantation workers an iron supplement. But an anthropologist familiar with the area—"and I guess I can say now it was my mother," Scrimshaw confides—disagreed. "Women got up before the men to prepare meals and look after children, went to the fields and did the same work as men, returned home to tend children, kitchen gardens and small animals raised for food and income, and were also responsible for purchasing food and keeping the house clean," she goes on. "Often, all of this was done while pregnant and lactating. The men rose later in the morning, had fewer family-related chores and rested in the evening after work."[6]

"If anyone needed that iron supplementation, it was the women," she goes on. "What's more, the men and women had different spending patterns for income. Women were more likely to put extra money into food or books or clothes for children; men were more likely to spend money on alcohol or something like a radio. The assumption that additional income produced by men would automatically go into children's mouths was incorrect."[7] Studies in other countries find similar results.

Many cultures prescribe special eating patterns during such nutritionally sensitive—yet spiritually or socially powerful—periods as menstruation, pregnancy, and nursing, whether to protect the community at large from the spiritual danger of menstrual blood or to ensure a healthy child. In some places, menstruating or expectant women are forbidden to cook or to eat certain foods. In others, they get special helpings of highly nourishing treats. And following birth, Scrimshaw notes, "in many cultures, female infants and children receive less food, less health care and less attention."[8] Such early deprivation, of course, often results in the problems of bone structure, pelvic development, anemia and the like, that take such a toll during childbirth and in later life.

American girls, of course, generally need not worry about an actual physical scarcity of food, or about disease and poverty leaving them too weak and depleted to grow and function at their best. But poverty is not the only social force that can deprive people of the nourishment they need. From the time an American female begins putting on the fat that heralds her coming reproductive powers, from the time she begins to think about herself in relation to the opposite sex, the culture around her insists that an attractive female must be thin. For many women, this demand lasts at least through the end of their reproductive years. And all too often, it translates into a mandate to scant on sensible nutrition.

Two or three generations ago, this pressure was less intense. Curves were the fashion; men hankered after a shapely "broad" who met that description in various strategic locations. But the prepubescent contours of today's top fashion models and film stars contrast startlingly with the amplitude of erstwhile sex goddesses like Marilyn Monroe and Sofia Loren, not to mention the "sweater girls" and pinups who tantalized GIs during the 1940s. Over recent decades, though everyday Americans' average weight has in fact risen, the celluloid and video ideal of feminine beauty has shrunk to a standard of slimness utterly unattainable by the great majority of ordinary people.

But genetic and nutritional impossibility cannot dissuade large numbers of girls and women, especially in the teens and twenties, from striving for the approved degree of stylish emaciation. Such unrealistic images produce a situation that would be ridiculous were it not so dangerous. Not only are about one-fourth of all adult Americans trying to lose weight, but so are about 11% of those who consider their weight "about right" and even 4% of those who think themselves underweight.

This last, and most troubling, group of dieters—a likely source of future eating disorder victims—increased fivefold just between 1985 and 1990.[9] A substantial number of women at or slightly above their ideal weight are "obsessed with dieting and weight loss," says IOM's Committee to Develop Criteria for Evaluating the Outcomes of Approaches to Prevent and Treat Obesity. Cultural dictates, the committee believes, fuel "the current emphasis on thinness in this and many other [affluent] countries," mainly among women, and help to shape the attitudes of both genders.[10]

These pressures convince many, especially adolescent girls, to put their figure ahead of their future needs. Eating habits may well be worst during life's second decade, but some important nutritional demands, most particularly for calcium, are especially high. Though American men generally get enough of this bone-building mineral, most women get less than the recommended dietary allowance, especially during the prime bone-building years between puberty and 30. "Unfortunately, many female teenagers are more concerned about having thin thighs than adequate calcium and prefer to drink a diet cola" rather than a glass of milk, Barrett-Connor laments.[11]

Indeed, getting adequate nutrition while keeping weight low can take careful planning of a kind not encouraged by media advertising that simultaneously pushes both high-fat fast foods and snacks and low-calorie, artificially sweetened diet foods. Studies of military women, for example, mostly young and, if anything, more physically fit than their civilian counterparts, highlight the difficulty. For those who have chosen a career in the armed services, "body weight and thinness mean more than just aesthetics and health," write Colonel Karen Fridlund of the Office of the Surgeon General and colleagues.[12] Meeting specified weight limits for one's gender is a prerequisite for continuing a career. As only about half of Army women studied exercise three or more times a week, diet appears their main method of weight control.

Many soldiers get most or all of their food through Army rations, which, in their various freshly cooked, "pre-plated," and freeze-dried versions, are designed to provide the Military Recommended Daily Allowances. The prescribed quantities of certain nutrients exceed the civilian standard to allow for soldiers' greater physical activity. Military males generally appear able to meet these goals within a calorie supply that maintains their weight.

Whether in uniform or out, though, women generally eat less than men, even of their own height or weight. Studies have therefore found Army women falling short in needed energy, protein, and, like their civilian sisters generally, calcium and iron. Indeed, Fridlund and colleagues speculate that, as the rations now stand, women would have to eat almost 30% more calories than necessary to maintain their weight in order to get their full recommended supply of those two minerals exclusively from food.[13] Considering that soldiers eat meals professionally designed to provide adequate nutrition, and probably much better balanced than young Americans would pick on their own, the chances that a young woman who chooses her own food could do any better are small indeed.

So while women in many foreign countries struggle daily just to get enough to eat, and while dietary deficiencies account for many deaths from childbirth and disease in developing countries around the world, Americans worry not about under- but overconsuming calories, not about malnutrition but about overweight. And though some of this worry, especially among the young, involves frivolous concerns about appearance, much of it, especially as women age, involves far more serious considerations of health. Obesity has in fact been described as "the single most prevalent nutrition problem in the United States."[14]

A WEIGHTY PROBLEM

"Life in the United States is conducive to obesity," is a truth obvious not only to the obesity committee, but also to anyone who examines the statistics showing that Americans are fatter and heavier than ever before.[15] According to some counts, fully 35% of women and 31% of men older than 20 fall into the category of obese.[16] But while all authorities agree that excessive heft carries significant health hazards, not everyone agrees on how to define it.

"Overweight" and "obese" both describe people who tip the scales at higher than the recommended poundage for their height and build. In common parlance, the former denotes the person a bit above the mark and the latter a person extremely so. Strictly speaking, however, the terms do not occupy a single continuum. In technical language, someone is overweight if he weighs too much and obese if his body contains too much fat. Usually, of course, these conditions go hand in hand, but one can and sometimes does exist without the other. A zealous body builder, for example, might carry a good number of extra pounds as solid muscle. An inactive "couch potato" or an elderly person, on the other hand, may be simultaneously thin and flabby. "For practical purposes, however," concludes the committee, "most overweight people are also obese."[17] But, as if to exemplify the general interchangeability of the terms, the committee itself chooses to use the term "obesity" "consistently in referring to the condition of excess body weight."[18]

If defining the word requires precision, deciding exactly whom it applies to involves even finer distinctions and sometimes complicated methodology. The several available methods for gauging body fat, which include underwater weighing, measuring the thickness of skin folds, using dual-energy X-ray absorptiometry, and sending a tiny electric current through a person's body for bioelectric impedance analysis often require skilled examiners using sophisticated equipment. When these anthropometric tests are used, men and women are usually considered obese at 25 and 30% body fat, respectively.[19]

But the two most popular methods of determining overweight use mathematical comparisons of weight and height. Weight-for-height tables have been compiled from information on millions of individuals by both insurance companies like Metropolitan Life, whose 1959 and 1983 efforts remain in wide use, and the federal government, which issued its own in 1990. Various versions of such tables have come under attack for specifying weight categories too wide or too narrow, too heavy or too light, or permitting or not permitting weight to creep up toward middle age. Another widely used indicator, the body mass index (BMI), is popular in research and health care. It divides a person's weight in kilograms by the square of his height in meters. Thus, $BMI = kg/m^2$. The values are ordinarily presented in tables that can also be translated into inches and pounds. (See Table 7-2.)

Ascertaining an individual's proportion of fat is complicated, whatever method is used. But figuring out when that number becomes a potential health problem is more complicated still. In 1993 the NIH National Task Force on Prevention and Treatment of Obesity pegged that threshold at a BMI of 25 or more through age 34 and at 27 for ages

TABLE 7-2 Body Weight (in pounds) According to Height (in inches) and Body Mass Index

| | | | | | | | | Body Mass Index | | | | | | | | |
Height	19	20	21	22	23	24	25	26	27	28	29	30	31	32	33	34
							Body Weight									
58	91	95	100	105	110	114	119	124	129	133	138	143	148	152	157	162
59	94	99	104	109	114	119	124	129	134	139	144	149	154	159	164	169
60	97	102	107	112	117	122	127	132	138	143	148	153	158	163	168	173
61	101	106	111	117	122	127	132	138	143	148	154	159	164	169	175	180
62	103	109	114	120	125	130	136	141	147	152	158	163	168	174	179	185
63	107	113	119	124	130	135	141	147	152	158	164	169	175	181	186	192
64	111	117	123	129	135	141	146	152	158	164	170	176	182	187	193	199
65	114	120	126	132	138	144	150	156	162	168	174	180	186	192	198	204
66	118	124	131	137	143	149	156	162	168	174	180	187	193	199	205	212
67	121	127	134	140	147	153	159	166	172	178	185	191	198	204	210	217
68	125	132	139	145	152	158	165	172	178	185	191	198	205	211	218	224
69	128	135	142	149	155	162	169	176	182	189	196	203	209	216	223	230
70	133	140	147	154	161	168	175	182	189	196	203	210	217	224	231	237
71	136	143	150	157	164	171	179	186	193	200	207	214	221	229	236	243
72	140	148	155	162	170	177	185	192	199	207	214	221	229	236	244	251
73	143	151	158	166	174	181	189	196	204	211	219	226	234	241	249	257
74	148	156	164	171	179	187	195	203	210	218	226	234	242	249	257	265
75	151	159	167	175	183	191	199	207	215	223	231	239	247	255	263	271
76	156	164	172	181	189	197	205	214	222	230	238	246	255	263	271	279

continued on next page

TABLE 7-2 Continued

Height	Body Mass Index															
	35	36	37	38	39	40	41	42	43	44	45	46	47	48	49	50
	Body Weight															
58	167	172	176	181	186	191	195	200	205	210	214	219	224	229	233	238
59	174	179	184	188	193	198	203	208	213	218	223	228	233	238	243	248
60	178	183	188	194	199	204	209	214	219	224	229	234	239	244	250	255
61	185	191	196	201	207	212	217	222	228	233	238	244	249	254	260	265
62	190	196	201	206	212	217	223	228	234	239	245	250	255	261	266	272
63	198	203	209	214	220	226	231	237	243	248	254	260	265	271	277	282
64	205	211	217	223	228	234	240	246	252	258	264	269	275	281	287	293
65	210	216	222	228	234	240	246	252	258	264	270	276	282	288	294	300
66	218	224	230	236	243	249	255	261	268	274	280	286	292	299	305	311
67	223	229	236	242	248	255	261	268	274	280	287	293	299	306	312	319
68	231	238	244	251	257	264	271	277	284	290	297	304	310	317	323	330
69	236	243	250	257	263	270	277	284	290	297	304	311	317	324	331	338
70	244	251	258	265	272	279	286	293	300	307	314	321	328	335	342	349
71	250	257	264	271	279	286	293	300	307	314	321	329	336	343	350	357
72	258	266	273	281	288	295	303	313	317	325	332	340	347	354	362	369
73	264	272	279	287	294	302	309	317	324	332	340	347	355	362	370	377
74	273	281	288	296	304	312	319	327	335	343	351	358	366	374	382	390
75	279	287	294	302	310	318	326	334	342	350	358	366	374	382	390	398
76	287	296	304	312	320	328	337	345	353	361	370	378	386	394	402	411

SOURCE: Institute of Medicine, *Weighing the Options: Criteria for Evaluating Weight-Management Programs*, 1995, Table 2-1, pp. 41–42.

beyond that, basing its decision on studies correlating weight and health in various populations. Other authorities disagree, however, arguing that weight gain with age is not necessarily either acceptable or desirable.[20]

The National Center for Health Statistics, on the other hand, takes a somewhat different approach, eschewing the term "obesity" altogether. It distinguishes "overweight" and "extreme overweight," using the 85th and 95th percentiles, respectively, of 20- to 29-year-olds measured in the 1976-1980 Second National Health and Nutrition Examination Survey (NHANES II). These cutpoints correspond to BMIs of 27.8 and 31.1 for men and 27.3 and 32.3 for women and are based on population distributions and not health experience.[21]

NHANES III, completed in 1994, provides the most up-to-date figures available on the American physique. Information collected between 1988 and 1991 is now available and finds, by NCHS standards for BMI, a whopping 33% of men and women over 20 overweight and 14% severely so.[22] Both of these figures represent increases over previous surveys, and a 36% increase in just under 30 years.[23] People in nearly all age categories are getting heavier.[24] (See Table 7-3.)

We Americans generally gain weight as we age; among women, overweight is commonest between 50 and 59. More women than men of every race register as overweight, although the gender differential among whites is only about half of a percentage point, between 31.6% of men and 32.1% of women. Just under half of African American and Mexican-American women fall into the category of overweight, however, exceeding their men by about 17 and 8 percentage points, respectively. In certain age groups, as many as 80% of African Americans, Native Americans, Pacific Islanders, and Hispanics are overweight or obese.[25]

These apparent racial differences, however, may really represent sociology and culture rather than genes. In general, the poorer and less educated weigh more, a correlation especially strong among women. Only 29% of Americans who have been to college are overweight, as opposed to 36% of the high school graduates and 39% of those with less than a high school diploma.[26] Indeed, some studies suggest that African American and white women hold somewhat different views about weight, with African American women less concerned about being thin. The added stress of lower-class life could also make weight loss more difficult,

TABLE 7-3   Suggested Weights for Adults

Height[a]	Weight (pounds)[b]	
	19–34 Years Old	35 Years Old and Over
5'0"	97–128	108–138
5'1"	101–132	111–143
5'2"	104–137	115–148
5'3"	107–141	119–152
5'4"	111–146	122–157
5'5"	114–150	126–162
5'6"	118–155	130–167
5'7"	121–160	134–172
5'8"	125–164	138–178
5'9"	129–169	142–183
5'10"	132–174	146–188
5'11"	136–179	151–194
6'0"	140–184	155–199
6'1"	144–189	159–205
6'2"	148–195	164–210
6'3"	152–200	168–216
6'4"	156–205	173–222
6'5"	160–211	177–228
6'6"	164–216	182–234

NOTE: The higher weights in the ranges generally apply to men, who tend to have more muscle and bone; the lower weights more often apply to women, who have less muscle and bone.

[a]Without shoes.
[b]Without clothes.

SOURCE: Institute of Medicine, *Weighing the Options: Criteria for Evaluating Weight-Management Programs*, 1995, Table 2-2, page 45.

some observers believe.[27] Of course, as yet unknown metabolic differences among racial groups may also contribute.

If culture and values play such an important role, obesity is clearly a medical disorder unlike most others. "One remarkable feature of obesity is that its management requires a great deal of effort from the individual. Health-care providers or counselors can offer only advice and technical support at this time," the obesity committee notes.[28]

Neither the public nor the health profession expects people, through their own efforts and the exercise of will, to cure themselves of chronic diseases like diabetes or arthritis, nor would we blame them if they tried and failed. Only a small number of the extremely obese, however, are appropriate candidates for an effective medical intervention like gastric surgery. Available drugs, for example, are not generally considered safe for use over the long term. Stopping medication, moreover, often leads to gaining back the weight lost. For such an immensely common long-term condition, however, medical science provides not much more than counsel, chastisement, and encouragement. "There are few diseases in which health-care providers can offer so little for those who struggle so much," the obesity committee believes.[29]

Obesity is also unusual among medical conditions because "its victims suffer discrimination," the committee continues. "Perhaps most laypersons, health-care providers, and even obese individuals themselves do not perceive the metabolic nature of the disease and thus view obesity as a problem of willful misconduct—eating too much and exercising too little." Two out of three family doctors surveyed, for example, thought that obese people "lack self-control," and more than a third believed them "lazy." Third-year medical students expressed similar views, finding them "unpleasant, worthless, and bad."[30]

Clearly, though, it is our lack of knowledge about the condition's roots rather than the individuals struggling to overcome it that should be criticized. An obese person trying to control her weight faces "a continuous, lifelong struggle with no expectation that the struggle required will diminish with time," the committee believes. Even a temporary lapse brings immediate consequences.

Why should losing weight be such a struggle? For most of human history, and for many people even today, the ability—not to mention the opportunity—to put on extra pounds, far from posing a threat to health, was a priceless advantage in the fight for survival. We Americans generally live in a world of plentiful food and scant exercise. For most of humankind, life has always been the reverse: endless toil and unpredictable provisions.

Women, in particular, seem programmed to gain weight. Indeed, because bringing a healthy child to term takes 55,000 calories, and months or years of nursing takes scores of thousands more, the species' very survival has depended in large measure on women's ability to sock away energy in the form of adipose tissue.[31] Among less affluent peoples, ample feminine dimensions connote health, prosperity, and fertility, in short, the presumed ability to sustain a pregnancy regardless of the vagaries of harvest or hunt. Indeed, no girl can menstruate unless and until her body attains a sufficient ratio of fat to lean. When women become too thin, whether because of famine, athletic training, or anorexia, their periods simply stop. Over the past 100 or more years, improving diets and, possibly, reduced exercise—either or both of which could produce larger, heavier girls—appear to account for the 3-year drop in the average age of menarche (to the middle of the thirteenth year) between the early decades of the last century and the middle of this.[32]

MOTHERS OF RETENTION

This close and specifically female tie between fat and fertility lies at the root of what many women consider their basic weight problem, the time they spent bearing and nursing their children. Nutrition and weight become literally vital issues during pregnancy. Too little weight gain can, as both medical and lay people have long understood, make the difference between safety and danger, between health and sickness, and, sometimes, between life and death, for both mother and child.

It has been obvious since ancient times that a woman's ability to nourish her baby both in the womb and at the breast essentially determines his chances of survival. What has been much less clear is what childbearing and nursing mean to the mother's own long-term well-being. Until very recently, in fact, both clinicians and researchers have considered nutrition during and after pregnancy essentially as it affects the infant and the birth. Preparing its 1991 report, for example, IOM's Subcommittee on Nutrition During Lactation could locate "no studies that evaluated the effects of maternal nutrition on long-term outcomes related to lactation." It did, however, find the reason for this astounding omission, as well as for the "lack of interest in maternal outcomes" in general, to be "unclear."[33] It is clear, however, that extremely obvious, even elementary, questions about the consequences of childbearing for the mother have remained unanswered and, until the past decade or so, essentially unasked.

The mother nourishes the fetus exclusively from her own body. What she eats, doctors have long known, therefore figures importantly in fetal growth. But the baby's size figures just as crucially in both mother's and baby's chances of not dying in childbirth. In an age when maternal death is a rarity and safe cesareans commonplace, we need an effort of imagination to recall that, for the overwhelming bulk of the human experience, and in some places to this day, pregnancy and delivery took a woman through a passage fraught with mortal peril. Shakespeare portrayed an adult who had survived being "from his mother's womb untimely ripp'd"—as had Macbeth's nemesis, Macduff—as so surpassingly uncommon that his identity became the hinge on which the great tragedy's plot turned.

Only in recent generations has such an operation ceased to be a desperate last resort that generally ended in catastrophe for mother, child, or both. And one of the commonest situations requiring this drastic intervention was a baby too large to pass through his mother's birth canal. Until the early twentieth century, therefore, doctors seeking easier and safer deliveries restricted the mother's diet to keep the fetal weight down. The first published study on the subject, appearing in 1901, in fact noted that limiting a pregnant woman's intake could drop her baby's birth weight by 400 to 500 grams.[34]

By the 1920s, however, with medical care and maternal survival improving, doctors began to consider that the mother's weight gain also related to the baby's growth, indeed, that her weight gain could serve to indicate her—and, presumably, the baby's—state of nutrition. Studies definitely proved a connection between the amount of weight she gained and the baby's size at birth. Doctors now began to routinely track mothers' weight, paying more attention to excess rather than inadequate poundage. The former, they believed, indicated a risk of toxemia and its potentially fatal consequences. Avoiding salt became a common tactic for controlling gain, which doctors advised should amount to no more than 15 pounds altogether. On average, according to studies published in the late 1930s and early 1940s, women put on only about 20 pounds.[35]

By the early 1970s, however, researchers were convinced that a larger gain, 27.5 pounds, represented the "physiological normality" for a healthy young woman carrying her first pregnancy. They also believed that the mother's weight both before and during pregnancy exerted separate, but cumulative, influences on the baby's weight at birth. Heavier women who also put on considerable weight during pregnancy bore bigger babies than did thin women who put on a similar number of pounds.[36]

During the mid-1970s, constituent bodies of the Food and Nutrition Board, the American College of Obstetricians and Gynecologists, and the American Dietetic Association all recommended 20 to 25 pounds as the desirable range, to go on pretty steadily from the thirteenth week onward, ideally between 2.2 pounds (1 kilogram) and 6.6 pounds for each of the last 6 months.[37] By the late 1970s, textbooks were suggesting an end to weight limits and, within reason, permission for women to eat what they wanted. It also became clear that gestational weight gain should bear some relationship to a mother's weight before conception, with thinner women being advised to gain more. Over the past half century, in short, the recommended gain has essentially doubled, from 15 to about 30 pounds.[38]

That figure of 30 pounds is merely an average, however. Studying a group of women who gave birth to healthy babies, "you see that the range of weight gains was quite broad," King says; "a few women didn't gain any weight at all and as many as 5 percent gained over 51 pounds." The largest single group put on between 26 and 30 pounds, but they made up only 20% of participants.[39] In the heterogeneous American population, no one recommendation can serve for everyone. Many factors, including age and ethnic background, determine the weight gain appropriate for a given individual. For example, African Americans need to gain more than whites on average to bear babies of the same weight, and girls who become pregnant within a year or two of menarche need to gain more than girls who are older. Obese women, on the other hand, might do well to gain less because they have higher rates of complicated births and infant mortality than women of normal weight or below.[40]

Weight gain depends largely on how much a woman eats. Equally crucial to her own and her baby's health, however, is exactly what constitutes that intake. Studies have consistently shown that pregnant Americans average less than the Recommended Daily Allowances of eight important nutrients: vitamins B_6, D, E, and folate; calcium, iron, magnesium, and zinc.[41] Adequate iron is particularly crucial to safe delivery, and, as we have seen, anemia is a major cause of maternal death worldwide. Discouragingly, though, research in Europe shows that, in the pregnancy committee's words, "women in industrialized countries often cannot meet their iron needs from diet alone."[42]

Expectant mothers and their doctors thus face an important question: should they make up these nutritional deficiencies with supplements? Though supplementation can solve one problem, it can cause another: in large quantities, minerals such as iron, selenium, and zinc, and vitamins including A, B_6, C, and D can prove toxic to the fetus. As science cannot predict how much of a given substance consumed by the mother will cross the placenta to the fetus, experts advise that a carefully planned diet be the main source of nutrition. All pregnant Americans, however, need to receive iron in supplementary form, and appropriate amounts of B_6 have recently been shown to guard against the neural tube defects responsible for spina bifida and hydrocephalus.

Given the centrality of an adequate diet to a healthy mother and child, the fate of poorly nourished women and those lacking the means to buy proper food becomes all the more crucial. In 1974, the U.S. Department of Agriculture's Special Supplemental Food Program for Women, Infants and Children (WIC) began to provide low-income mothers and their children food packages and vouchers as well as nutrition education and counseling. Studies show that WIC participants get substantially more of the nourishment they need than comparable women who do not participate.[43]

The WIC program strives to give women who face special nutritional problems the knowledge and wherewithal to eat properly. And that, experts believe, should be the care provider's goal for every expectant mother. Early and adequate prenatal care becomes an absolute necessity if, as King recommends, all expectant mothers are to "receive an assessment of their dietary practices" and requirements in time to make a difference. Particular attention should go to "screening for women who may have problems relating to their lifestyle."[44] These include smoking, drug abuse, previous extreme dieting for weight loss, multiple pregnancies, and pica, the practice of eating nonfood substances such as laundry starch. Such an assessment can determine both the amount of weight an individual might sensibly gain and whether she needs any special dietary supplements.

NURSING MOTHERS

Only a minority of American mothers breastfeed for any substantial amount of time. Although experts now recommend mother's milk as the optimal food for all infants, just over half of new mothers undertake to nurse their newborns. After five or six months, fewer than half of those who started, and under one-fifth of all mothers, are still feeding their babies at the breast. Nor do the mothers who nurse represent a cross section of the nation. Twice as many married mothers as unmarried breastfeed, nearly twice as many whites as African Americans, and nearly twice as many residents of the mountain and West Coast states as of the Southeast. (See Figures 7-1 and 7-2.) The more educated a woman and the higher her family income, the more likely she is not only to begin breastfeeding but also to persevere.[45]

Breastfeeding has not always been the choice of the nation's best informed and most affluent, however. Early in the twentieth century, as is still true today, sophisticated people who kept up with scientific developments overwhelmingly chose the latest in nutritional methods. These individuals of course included independent-minded women who sought broader career horizons than their old-fashioned mothers. For many of our mothers and grandmothers, the most up-to-date choice was feeding their babies formula from bottles. At a time when the promise of better infant survival rates was becoming real, making sure that a baby got the proper amount of milk seemed rational and prudent. At a time when only those wealthy enough to afford wet nurses could avoid nursing their children at their own breasts, breastfeeding symbolized not the most forward-looking nutritional and ecological awareness but an apparently outmoded domesticity. Thus, as the newer, more "scientific" bottlefeeding method spread from the opinion-making elite to the broader public, the percentage of American women breastfeeding fell through most of this century. About three-quarters of babies born in the late 1930s were nursed. By the early 1970s the number was under one-quarter.[46]

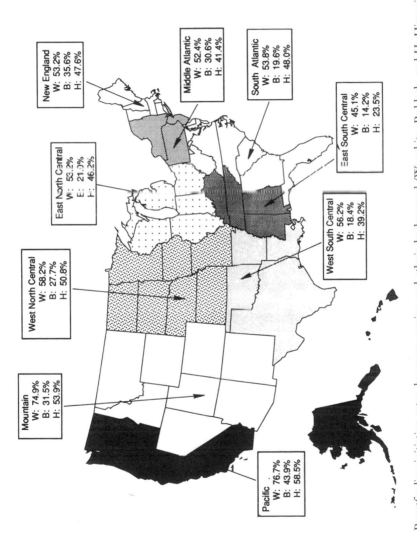

New England
W: 53.2%
B: 35.6%
H: 47.6%

Middle Atlantic
W: 52.4%
B: 30.6%
H: 41.4%

South Atlantic
W: 53.8%
B: 19.6%
H: 48.0%

East South Central
W: 45.1%
B: 14.2%
H: 23.5%

East North Central
W: 53.2%
B: 21.9%
H: 46.2%

West South Central
W: 56.2%
B: 18.4%
H: 39.2%

West North Central
W: 58.2%
B: 27.7%
H: 50.8%

Mountain
W: 74.9%
B: 31.5%
H: 53.9%

Pacific
W: 76.7%
B: 43.9%
H: 58.5%

FIGURE 7-1 Breastfeeding initiation rates, by census region and ethnic background (W: white, B: black, and H: Hispanic). SOURCE: *Nutrition During Lactation*, Institute of Medicine, 1991, Figure 3-2, page 34.

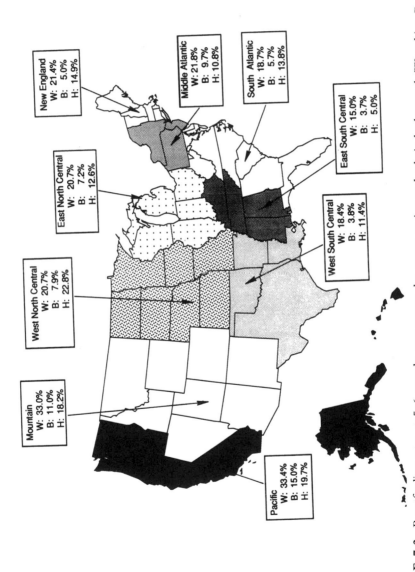

FIGURE 7-2 Breastfeeding rates at 5–6 months postpartum, by census region and ethnic background (W: white, B: black, and H: Hispanic). SOURCE: *Nutrition During Lactation*, Institute of Medicine, 1991, Figure 3–3, page 35.

By the middle of the 1970s, however, a new understanding of breast milk's unique benefits began changing mothers' opinions and feeding habits, again with the best-off and best educated leading the way toward apparently new and apparently more natural methods, such as breastfeeding. During this same period, natural childbirth—a return to delivery with a minimum of anesthetic—also returned to favor, ousting the more aggressive anesthetic and surgical methods that had earlier seemed to be the ultimate in medical progress.

The advantages of breastfeeding derive, of course, from the fact that, because the food comes from the mother's own body, it matchlessly suits the infant who receives it. But that advantage also means that the milk's constituents can come only from either the mother's food supply or her own body's stores of nutrients. Because research has concentrated overwhelmingly on the supply and composition of the milk—in other words, on the baby's needs rather than the mother's experience—"the nutritional status of lactating women has not been thoroughly or extensively studied," the lactation subcommittee notes.[47]

It does appear that well-nourished American women generally have no difficulty providing their babies ample nutrition. Nursing demands about 640 calories per day, more than twice the 300 needed each day to support the last six months of pregnancy.[48] A daily 2,700 calories rich in sources of calcium, protein, vitamins, and minerals appears to supply essentially all the nutrients a woman needs both to nourish her baby and to sustain or replenish her own body's stores of nutrients, with the possible exception of calcium and zinc. If her diet falls much below that calorie level, however, or if it is substantially less nutritious than the average American intake, she will most likely lack other vitamins and minerals as well.[49] The nursing mothers most at risk for eating poorly belong, not surprisingly, to those groups who generally eat poorly in any case: young adolescents, especially those of poor families; African American women; and the poor. Here, again, the WIC program can make a major difference.

THE LONG RUN

Of all that science does not yet know about maternal nutrition during pregnancy and lactation, perhaps the least known and least studied aspect is what they ultimately do to the mother's body. The large supplies of nutrients as well as the drastic adjustments needed to nourish an embryo from a single cell to a 7- or 8-pound newborn and then to feed that baby while he doubles his weight in the first 4 to 6 months "involve nearly every maternal organ system," according to the lactation subcommittee.[50] And increasing evidence suggests that, in case a mother's supply proves inadequate to satisfy them both, the baby's needs often take precedence over her own, stripping her own stores to supply him. A poorly nourished woman thus grows her baby in part at her own body's expense.

But we do not know what specifically this drain of calories, minerals, and other substances does to even a healthy, well-nourished mother over the long term. A woman bestows about 30 grams of calcium on her baby during pregnancy, for example, and another 8 to 10 grams during each month she nurses. A woman weighing in the range of 120 pounds thus provides 3% of her own body's total calcium before her baby is even born and another 5% by the time she has nursed for 6 months. Some evidence exists—from animal rather than human studies, however— that her ability to absorb calcium from food may rise during lactation. But even so, replacing what she loses means consuming hundreds of milligrams each day on top of the 1,000 daily milligrams recommended to all women.[51,52]

Does this massive calcium transfer contribute to later osteoporosis? "Data suggest that acute bone loss is likely to occur during lactation," the subcommittee notes, but studies also indicate that the metabolism of bone changes to accommodate these tremendous demands without devastating the mother's skeleton. Some researchers even deem it likely that breastfeeding may hasten the deposition of calcium in at least some of the mother's bones. And studies have found higher bone mass among postmenopausal white women who had nursed than among those who had not. But the evidence about a possible relationship between the vital female function of nourishing one's children and one of the most prevalent feminine diseases of later life remains, in the subcommittee's words, "inconclusive."[53]

The other big reproductive question weighing, as it were, on women's minds is the connection between pregnancy, lactation, and obesity. Here there is a body of research, and, alas, it does confirm "women's sense that overweight in mid-life is related to reproductive events," says Kathleen Maher Rasmussen, Sc.D., R.D., professor of nutritional sciences at Cornell. Women "weigh more and are fatter after delivery than they were at conception." The more pounds a pregnant mother puts on before birth, the more she will take off afterward, but the more she will also weigh when next she conceives.[54]

Lactation, however, takes off pounds and fat. Mother rats, at least, are leaner when they finish nursing than they were when they conceived. Whether the same goes for women is not yet clear. Those studied, generally college-educated whites, lose, on average, a pound or two a month for the first half year or so they nurse.[55] The loss continues in later months, but its rate slows. But women who nurse differ systematically from the general population, and the nature of that differentness has changed over recent decades, facts that considerably complicate the statistics of recent research. And since rats all nurse for essentially the same amount of time, and never supplement their babies' diets with bottles or foods, their experience makes them far more uniform research subjects than human mothers, who nurse as long and as often as they wish and feed their children whatever else they please on the side.

This and just about every other aspect of human reproduction is now discretionary, in this country at least. Women thus have "choices about how much they will weigh at mid-life," Rasmussen believes, and several of the most important have to do with reproduction. The 2 pounds or so that two or three children will add, on average, to their mother's figure probably will not weigh heavily in her decision making. But more children than that may add a considerably larger amount of cumulative poundage. Thus, staying at the low end of the recommended weight gain range in each pregnancy might save her five or more retained pounds. Deciding to breastfeed will also help her get back to where she started, especially if she watches her calories during the time she nurses.[56]

THE LATER YEARS

What she ate and did in earlier decades has obviously already said a good deal about a woman's health before she passes into the last third of her life. Her peak bone density, determined by the calcium she ate or did not eat while young, is already a decade or two in the past. Her chances of breast and other reproductive cancers may well depend in part on the fat content of long-ago meals.

But that is not to say that what she eats day to day does not still play a crucial role in maintaining her well-being. The question now becomes not so much "how we can achieve a longer life, although that would be nice," says Irwin Rosenberg, M.D., director of the U.S. Department of Agriculture's Human Nutrition Research Center on Aging at Tufts University, "but the quality of life and the maintenance of a high degree of activity and the prevention of disability"—factors that, as we have seen, determine a woman's ability to remain independent and involved in old age. "And there is where I think the nutrition and health nexus is particularly important."[57]

Though an older woman can no longer affect the maximum mineral density of her bones, she can do a good deal to preserve the bone mass she has. In addition to calcium, vitamin D appears crucial to the state of the older skeleton, although blood levels of the vitamin tend to drop with age. Between the twenties and the eighties, a person's skin loses as much as 60% of its ability to synthesize this vitamin in sunlight. The intestines also lose some of their ability to absorb it from food. With less of the vitamin available from former sources, studies show that supplementation can help preserve women's mineral density, making vitamin D a "compelling" issue in the question of how to retain bone mass, Rosenberg believes.[58]

Adequate levels of other vitamins may also help preserve other crucial capacities. As the body's ability to absorb vitamin B_{12} drops, especially in the presence of certain stomach conditions, so may cognitive function. Supplementation, however, may counteract this trend. Adequate supplies of zinc and B_6 may slow the decline in immune function. And vitamin C may be useful in preventing cataracts, half again as common in women as in men.[59]

These problems with vitamins are only some of the bodily changes that make the later years nutritionally challenging. Indeed, at a time when a woman needs more of certain nutrients in her diet than ever before, her body conspires to make her need less food over all. Not only are the bones thinning and the fat layer thickening, but an individual's lean body mass declines with age and the muscle mass declines even more dramatically. With the drop in lean tissue, and especially in muscles, the person's daily caloric requirement also falls at the rate of about 100 calories a decade. By the time it reaches 1,400 or 1,500 during the Social Security years, planning an adequately nutritious diet that does not put on weight becomes rather difficult. Exercise, which has been shown to build muscle even in a woman's tenth decade, thus becomes crucial to maintaining the muscle mass needed for both mobility and nutrition. It also enables a woman to consume more food without gaining weight, thereby improving her nutritional status if the choices are appropriate ones.

THE DIETER'S DILEMMA

Still, with culture and probably endocrinology and genetics against them, more Americans of all ages are dieting than ever before, spending billions of dollars each year on books, drugstore diet aids, special foods, and commercial weight loss programs, and the like, to shed unwanted pounds. Regardless of how they go about it, though, whether they join a support group or enroll in a commercial plan, whether they buy special foods or count their calories or fat grams, most Americans experience results that are, in the words of Judith Stern, Sc.D., professor of Nutrition at the University of California at Davis, "quite dismal." Even among those enrolling in obesity treatment programs, most "really don't lose significant weight permanently." According to one classic study, "about a third won't lose any weight, a third will lose significant amounts of weight, and a third will drop out." And over a period of years, even the big losers regain much or all of their hard-lost flab.[60]

That's because, even more dishearteningly, "based on scientific evidence, it appears that some obese people, when they reduce their weight, are not made normal by weight reduction."[61] They may, for example, have started out with more fat cells than thinner individuals. For them, losing weight merely reduces the size but not the number of "these cells waiting to be filled up" again, Stern notes. What's more, she adds, the enzyme lipoprotein lipase, present in fatty tissue, acts "as a gatekeeper enzyme to allow fat to enter the fat cell."[62] Obese individuals—and obese animals, too—have high levels of this enzymatic activity. It drops with their weight, but not to the levels typical of people of normal dimensions. Scientists speculate that the enzyme may thus ease the almost inevitable return of the unwanted pounds.

Given these discouraging realities, Stern believes, "it's no wonder that we rarely . . . design diets that effectively keep weight off forever. In addition, we don't really understand the fundamental causes of obesity, and obesity isn't a single disease."[63] That's why those dissatisfied with their figures face such a plethora of options: diets of every description, self-help organizations, commercial groups, over-the-counter drugs, medically supervised very-low-calorie diets and near-fasts, and, for the truly morbidly obese, surgery. These various methods combine limiting intake, usually by counting calories (800 to 1,200 daily in many low-calorie diets, below 800 daily in the very-low-calorie versions) or grams of fat; increasing physical activity, though this is often "an afterthought, rather than an integral part" of the program, according to the obesity committee[64]; behavior modification, such as trying to learn new habits through systems of rewards and self-monitoring; and medications that either dampen appetite or raise metabolism. Gastric surgery, appropriate only for certain very overweight individuals proven unable to control their obesity by conventional means, reshapes the stomach to limit intake.

"In this country, where successful weight management has proven an elusive goal for most obese individuals, the marketplace has provided many legitimate, as well as unfounded, products and services," the obesity committee warns. The latter operators "play legal tag with government regulatory agencies while taking financial advantage of a public desperate for answers. Improving the rate of success at weight management requires that would-be dieters understand that methods from thigh creams to esoteric diets must be substantiated by validated evidence of efficacy. They may represent no more than small countermeasures to an incompletely understood disorder of energy balance."[65]

Indeed, those people who do manage to lose weight and keep it off seem to use methods neither exotic nor extreme. A fundamental part of most successful programs is exercise, which not only burns calories but alters metabolism. It must remain a continuing part of the dieter's life, however, because ceasing to exercise regularly also changes metabolism, but in the wrong direction.

People who lose weight and maintain their loss are twice as likely as those who lose and then regain it to have designed their own programs. The details of each individual's private system—counting calories, cutting out certain categories of foods, keeping track of fats, adopting bits and pieces of various commercial methods—seem less important, Stern believes, than the fact that "it was the individual who took responsibility for the weight loss program, not the health care worker."[66]

Personal motivation and values are clearly central to successful diet control. In the Women's Health Trial, a precursor to WHI, women inspired by the possibility of reducing their known high risk for breast cancer succeeded in dropping their fat intake to a mere 20% of total calories—about half of the average American level—for an impressive 24 months. And they did it by revising their total eating habits. Their success, Henderson speculates, could highlight "an area in which there could be a distinct gender difference linked with the responsibility for providing food. It's so much easier to change food planning, purchasing and preparation, than exercising restraint at the table."[67]

And, indeed, men do generally choose a different approach to weight loss than do women, preferring exercise over dieting, the main female strategy. Also indicating the relationship of values and weight, white women appear to value weight loss somewhat more than African American women do. And lots of women, but many fewer men, who are not even overweight nonetheless actively diet. The effect of repeated cycles of loss and gain—so-called yo-yo dieting—on an individual's health and future ability to maintain a reasonable weight remains controversial. Some believe that severe dieting results in a lower basal metabolism at the end than at the beginning, as the body goes into a crisis mode to avoid starvation. Others disagree. But one type of dieter at least, the nonobese teenage girl, "should be actively discouraged," Stern notes, because "she may under some circumstances be setting herself up for obesity later on by depressing her basal metabolism."[68]

Clearly, of course, the best solution would be for all women to avoid becoming overweight in the first place. Studies of both women who never gained excessively and those who lost weight and kept it off revealed an activist attitude, both toward keeping track of their weight and keeping physically active. Such women also took a more direct approach to daily problems and stress than women who lost weight but relapsed into obesity.[69]

While government goals for the turn of the century call for no more than 20% of adults and 15% of adolescents to be obese, our nation's efforts to shape up have not met with conspicuous success. And our national experience with smoking ought to encourage skepticism that deeply ingrained behaviors are anything but extremely difficult to change. Still, "the most optimistic feature" of this situation lies in the promise of current and future research, the obesity committee believes. "Learning more about how health-related behaviors develop and can be modified, together with the rapid growth of knowledge and better tools in areas such as molecular genetics and metabolic regulation, gives promise that at some point we will understand the underlying causes of obesity. This should ultimately lead to the development of programs that treat the underlying causes of obesity and not just the symptoms."[70]

But we need not wait for these important discoveries to be realized before we adopt a far healthier attitude toward weight and nutrition. "Many people are obsessed with their weight in a culture that encourages one both subtly and overtly to equate thinness with beauty and obesity with sloth," the committee continues. Rather, the goal for everyone, regardless of their weight, age, or gender, should be to adopt a diet that maximizes health. For those whom overweight threatens to harm, the obesity committee advises the goal of weight management, which, in contrast to mere weight loss, judges eating and other habits "more by their effects on the overall health of participants than by their effects on weight alone."[71]

If every woman in America adopted this attitude, and the eating pattern it implies, if we could break the tyranny of thinness and refocus on physical and mental well-being, then young girls would not starve themselves in the cause of fashion, mothers and babies would receive the nutrition they need, and the rates of chronic diseases in the later years would fall. By "eating for life" rather than for appearance's sake, women can not only lengthen their lives but enrich them.

NOTES

1. Barrett-Connor (1991), 4.
2. Ibid., 7.
3. King (1991), 7.
4. Barrett-Connor (1991), 9.
5. Ibid., 27.
6. Scrimshaw (1991), 3.
7. Ibid., 4.
8. Ibid., 11.
9. *Weighing the Options: Criteria for Evaluating Weight-Management Programs*, 54.
10. Ibid.
11. Barrett-Connor (1991), 9.
12. Fridlund et al. (1991), 8.
13. Ibid., 22.
14. *Healthy People 2000: Citizens Chart the Course*, 112.
15. *Weighing the Options*, 134.
16. Ibid., 27.
17. Ibid., 40.
18. Ibid.
19. Ibid., 40.
20. Ibid., 44-5.
21. Ibid., 43.
22. Ibid., 47.
23. Ibid.
24. Ibid., 47-8.
25. Ibid., 128.
26. Ibid., 126.
27. Ibid., 129.
28. Ibid., 38.
29. Ibid., 39.
30. Ibid.
31. *Nutrition During Pregnancy*, 169.
32. Ibid., 43.
33. *Nutrition During Lactation*, 196.
34. Ibid., 38.
35. Ibid.
36. Ibid.
37. Ibid., 39.
38. Ibid., 40.
39. King (1991), 4.
40. Ibid., 6.
41. *Nutrition During Pregnancy*, 269.
42. Ibid., 278.
43. Ibid., 269.
44. King (1991), 11.
45. *Nutrition During Lactation*, 33.
46. Ibid., 29, 30.
47. Ibid., 74.
48. Ibid., 213.

49. Ibid., 229.
50. Ibid., 197.
51. Ibid., 104.
52. *Eat for Life: The Food and Nutrition Board's Guide for Reducing Your Risk of Chronic Disease*, 21.
53. *Nutrition During Lactation*, 208.
54. Rasmussen (1991), 12.
55. *Nutrition During Lactation*, 74.
56. Rasmussen (1991), 14.
57. Rosenberg (1991), 3.
58. Ibid., 9.
59. Ibid., 12 , 13, 18.
60. Stern (1991), 2.
61. Ibid.
62. Ibid., 3.
63. Ibid., 2.
64. *Weighing the Options*, 83.
65. Ibid., 36.
66. Stern (1991), 8.
67. IOM 1992 Annual Meeting, 20.
68. Stern (1991), 20.
69. Ibid., 9.
70. *Weighing the Options*, 30.
71. Ibid., 131.

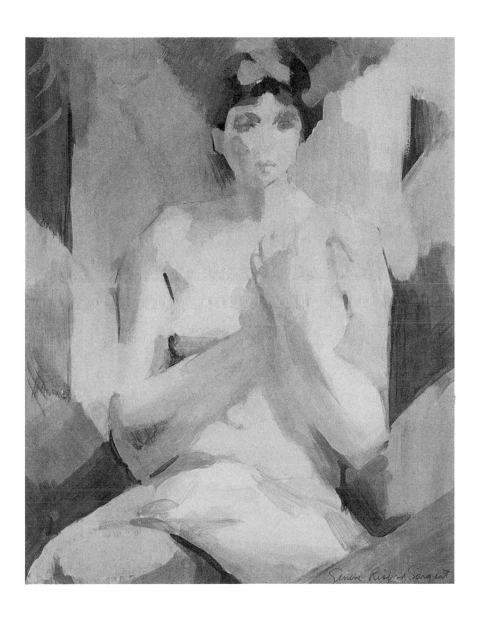

Geneve Rixford Sargeant
Portrait of Eleanor (1930)
Gouache on paper
The National Museum of Women in the Arts
Gift of Wallace and Wilhelmina Holladay

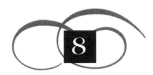

Women in the
Health Care System

The American health care system is a mass of contradictions. Our great medical centers boast the most sophisticated technologies, the most expert subspecialists, the most massive research enterprise the world has ever seen. Yet our people meanwhile suffer some of the worst rates of infant mortality and cervical cancer, among other preventable tragedies, in the industrialized world. Our talented medical professionals perform at the peak of their art while many ordinary citizens go without routine care. To paraphrase a famous World War II military motto, the difficult we do immediately. The simple takes a lot longer.

In this increasingly complicated system, women's health needs present an especially confusing picture. Biochemical wizardry allows babies to be conceived in the laboratory in the same country—indeed, sometimes in the same hospital—where women who have gone their entire pregnancy without seeing a doctor arrive unannounced in advanced labor. Teams of specialists transplant bone marrow in hopes of saving women from late-stage breast cancer at the same time that many other women have no access to the routine exams and mammography that could detect tumors in the more easily curable early stages.

This tangle of paradoxes permits few sweeping generalizations about the American experience of health care, except perhaps for this: in a number of significant ways, the system treats the genders differently.

Whether as patients or as health care providers, women function within it in a distinctively feminine fashion.

Differences show up most obviously, perhaps, in the health care professions. Large numbers of women now practice medicine, but men still predominate in such prestigious posts as those of professors and deans. Women throng the lesser-paying fields as nurses; allied health professionals like technicians, audiologists, and occupational therapists; and low-skilled workers like nurses aides and home health care aides. As patients seeking a doctor or trying to pay their bills, women also differ from men. They have specifically female patterns and needs, but the American health care system, like much else about the medical enterprise in the United States, still operates on a largely male model.

Most crucial from the patients' point of view, "men and women in the United States experience different access to health care," according to Nancy Anne Fugate Woods, Ph.D., professor of nursing and director of the Center for Women's Health Research at the University of Washington. Factors beyond most people's control decide who can get needed care and who cannot.[1] Do appropriate providers offer the right services at places and times the patient can get to? Do they have room for her in their schedules and practices? Will they accept her? Does she find the services acceptable? Can she pay for them? "Each of these factors is affected by gender," Woods notes.[2] Each plays out differently for males and females.

Women get sick more often than men, as we have already noted. Not surprisingly, they use health services more often and are more likely to seek them from a regular source of care; fully 84% of women, but only 75% of men, depend on a usual provider. And women's use of medical services follows a distinctive pattern. Until age 15 or so, girls and boys both see a pediatrician or family practitioner. For the next three decades, though, until the mid-forties, many women use an OB/GYN as their main medical advisor; men almost never get primary care from doctors who specialize in their reproductive system. Childbearing accounts for much of this difference, of course, and as women age their patterns again begin to more closely resemble men's. After menopause, they turn increasingly to family practitioners and internists.

Over their lifetime, women on average also spend more time

in hospitals, including psychiatric ones, where they account for a larger portion of inpatient admissions than men. Both genders need and use more medical care as they grow older. Regardless of age, though, the poor visit doctors less often than other Americans.[3]

But the fact that women make greater use of medical facilities does not guarantee that they get all the care or the kind of care they need. Bureaucratic arrangements and intellectual assumptions, many totally un-related to the real needs of real people, vastly complicate many women's quest for medical attention and deprive some of even rudimentary ser-vices. (Certain other aspects of the health care system, meanwhile, may have detrimental—though different—effects on certain men.) "Grounded in assumptions about men as normal and reproduction as a central aspect of women's health," Woods declares, "our current arrangements have created different access to health care for men and women and perpetu-ated an organization of health services that serves men's health care needs differently from those of women."[4]

GETTING WHAT ONE NEEDS

Central to any medical system is the basic question of whether people can get what they need when they need it. In this country, "money, time, and geography" determine the answer, according to Woods. Does a patient have a way of getting to a suitable facility at a time when it's offering service? Can she trust the quality of diagnosis and treatment? Can she afford to pay the bill? Women's experience differs from men's "in each of these dimensions," Woods notes, but finance "looms as the critical issue for the decade." As a group, women are far less able than men to pay for all the health care they need.[5]

One of the reasons is obvious: women simply earn less than men—72 cents for every male dollar in 1991, giving them less money to spend on both bills and insurance premiums.[6] More than three-quarters of all Americans—and a slightly higher percentage of women than men—nonetheless have some form of coverage. But women less often use pri-vate plans and more often depend on public assistance programs like Med-icaid, which drastically curtail options because many providers refuse publicly funded patients.[7]

Of America's 37 million uninsured, whose choices are even more drastically limited, 17 million are female. Of the women who have insurance, the youngest and oldest are less likely than average to hold private policies; those under 24 are least likely of all. Nearly all women over 65—95% to be exact—have Medicare, and 77% carry additional private coverage.[8]

Indeed, "the elderly enjoy better access to care, in the form of insurance coverage, than any other age group in the nation," found IOM's Panel on the National Health Care Survey in 1992. "By contrast, individuals and families with low incomes"—a group that includes millions of mothers and children—"are not well covered by the federal-state Medicaid program."[9] Women in the childbearing years face the highest risk of inadequate coverage, at a time in their lives when need is often acute. Later, between menopause and Medicare—the decades from 45 to 65—they are likelier than men to have no insurance at all. These uninsured come disproportionately from the ranks of minorities, the unemployed, and singles, whether divorced, widowed, or never married.[10]

A woman's chance of getting medical care thus depends crucially on her employment and marital status; she may often find herself disadvantaged compared to a comparable man. Fewer female workers get insurance as a job benefit, with the disproportionately female holders of part-time and unskilled jobs least likely to enjoy this valuable "perk." Even among the overwhelmingly female health care workforce, many employees lack health coverage. Some 6% of those staffing doctors' offices, for instance, have no health insurance, and 52% get no employer contribution toward their premiums.[11] And even in this age of two-paycheck families, many mothers still cut back their work hours or leave the labor force altogether, at least temporarily. A full-time mom thus usually finds herself at the mercy of her husband's insurance, assuming that she has a husband and he has insurance. Today's high divorce rate, however, along with the fact that 15% of employed workers' dependents lack coverage, renders both assumptions tenuous for many.[12]

But even if a woman does have private insurance, she still may face special disadvantages because a policy as good as a man's still may not protect her adequately. Plans providing the same benefits for both genders often leave women uncovered during the two periods when they need it most, the childbearing years and old age. In the reproductive decades, most policies disallow pregnancies conceived before beginning a job and many exclude cancer screening, pregnancy, delivery, postpartum care, and abortion services. (However, the recent Kennedy-Kassebaum Health Insurance Bill prohibits denying insurance coverage based on medical conditions.—ED.) More than 80% of family physicians offer family planning, but most private plans consider it unreimbursable preventive care, leaving patients to pay for office visits and birth control supplies out of their own pockets.

Poor women, of course, can resort to the nation's 5,000 family planning clinics, which together provide more than a third of total contraceptive services. But in public as well as private facilities, preventing a pregnancy and terminating it are two different stories. "In contrast to family planning services, abortion services are becoming less available to women," Woods notes, "even though the number of abortions performed remains relatively constant. Federal policy has left poor women without access to abortion care, and many private insurance carriers do not cover the service," which can cost between $300 and almost $2,000, depending on where and when it is performed. "The 1978 Pregnancy Discrimination Act permits abortion services to be excluded from coverage. To my knowledge, there is no other federal regulation that condones the exclusion of a health service to men."[13]

Then, in old age, Woods adds, women face the crushing costs of long-term care, whether in institutions or their own homes. Most policies, however, including Medicare, stress "acute care, such as hospitalization, emphasizing curative services more commonly needed by older men"—an oversight that pauperizes many old women. Overall, Woods concludes, omitting the services that women need most constitutes "unintended rationing of health care based on gender."[14]

Lack of child care during medical appointments and office or clinic hours that conflict with jobs and family responsibilities are among the more formidable nonfinancial obstacles. Indeed, women's very role as family nurturers, their "extra-market work as mothers, wives and informal caregivers paradoxically provides health care to others," Woods notes, but can prevent them from meeting their own needs. Although 82% provide an annual physical for their children, only 69% get one themselves.[15]

Further severe rationing occurs by race, income, and geography. "For poor patients, financial problems are exacerbated by the necessity of coping with lack of transportation, child care, and the ability to take time off from work," concurs a report by IOM's Committee on Monitoring Access to Personal Health Care Services.[16] In both city neighborhoods and rural counties across America, a severe shortage of doctors who accept Medicaid, or the total absence of any doctors at all, forces the ill and expectant to choose between long journeys and foregoing care altogether. More than 80% of America's counties, home to almost a third of reproductive-age women, lack any source of abortion services.[17]

Whether due to insufficient insurance or unmanageable logistics, inadequate access translates into needless suffering and death. People who cannot see a doctor, whatever the reason, miss the relatively cheap and simple preventive services and screenings that can forestall costly catastrophes like late-stage tumors and complicated births. Lack of prevention thus creates a deadly class discrepancy. Breast cancer strikes African American women less often than whites, for example—96.6 cases per 100,000 women as opposed to 112.9 per 100,000—but kills them more often—27 per 100,000 versus 23 per 100,000.[18] In poor areas, tumors are 20% more likely to have reached the lethal late stages by the time they are found than in more affluent locales. Over a period of 15 years, incidence of late-stage cancers fell by more than 21% in high-income communities but by only 6% in poorer ones.[19] Simply having mammograms and breast examinations boosts by 20% a woman's chance of living 5 years.[20]

"Although we can detect tumors as small as 3 to 5 milligrams with mammography, we continue to see too many large, clinically obvious carcinomas that carry a poor prognosis," says Valerie P. Jackson, M.D., of the Indiana University School of Medicine. "Noncompliance is a problem for all groups of women, but it is particularly prevalent in our elderly and indigent populations," many of whom cannot afford even $50 for a potentially life-saving mammogram.[21] Since Medicare now pays for screening (as opposed to just diagnostic) mammograms, cost should no longer be a deterrent and compliance should improve.

Another deadly malignancy, vastly simpler than breast cancer to prevent, detect, and cure, reveals even more disturbing inequities of access. Cervical cancer, though easily found in its early, and even precancerous, stages by the cheap and reliable Pap smear, strikes African American women twice as often as whites and kills them three times as often. Many of these deaths, and particularly the "excess" ones, reflect plain neglect. A Pap test even once every five years slashes mortality by 84%, once every two years by 93%. In the early 1970s, African Americans had largely lethal late-stage diagnoses about as often as whites, but twice as often by the late 1980s.[22] So large a "relative difference in late-stage cancer among different groups is an important clue to the existence of problems with access and, potentially, with subsequent treatment," notes the IOM committee on access.[23]

Nor is cancer screening the only routine care whose lack disproportionately kills poor and nonwhite Americans. In the late 1980s, a deadly venereal disease supposedly vanquished decades before began an ominous rise. The syphilis rate among African American adults more than doubled in only four years, and the congenital form—fatal almost half the time—began showing up in African American infants. "Fully preventable by treating infected women with penicillin early in pregnancy," this killer "should be a disease of the past," declares a 1990 editorial in the *American Journal of Public Health* cited by the access committee. Instead, as a "sentinel health condition" it marks a serious public health failure.[24]

Such a lapse entails more than poor financial or physical access, however. Even getting herself to a clinic or doctor's office provides a poor person no assurance of good-quality care. Fully three-quarters of the women who missed a mammogram during a two-year period had seen a doctor during that time. Many of those physicians failed to convey the test's life-and-death importance. For the access committee, such failures raise "the question of why the test was not performed during the visit and whether the barrier to screening here is one of poor-quality care rather than access to care."[25]

Part of the answer lies in where a woman gets her care, a factor that can strongly influence its quality. Fully 85% of health maintenance organization members get a timely Pap smear, as opposed to 75% of private physicians' patients. Only 58% of those without a regular health care source had the test in the past three years, usually at a public health or community clinic. Doctors' attitudes also partially explain the Pap gap. Many feel awkward "pressing poor patients to pay for and undergo screening procedures," the access committee found, "particularly if the patients were having difficulty paying their rent. Similarly, when a diabetic patient can barely afford the cost of medication, her physician may be reluctant to urge her to have a mammogram that is expensive and often not covered by insurance."[26]

Then there is the "reluctance of some physicians" to do screening procedures like Paps and breast exams because they feel "discomfort" or think that "these tests are best left to gynecologists"—specialists whom poor women are exceedingly unlikely to visit. "Internists and family practitioners, however, are specifically trained in these procedures during residency," the committee notes. Altogether, these "structural deficiencies in the organization of care" add up to access problems reaching far "beyond the usual financial limits."[27]

Similar sorts of structural barriers, including physician attitudes, in fact reach well beyond preventive care. "Battering," the access committee stated, "is a major factor in injury and illness among women"—indeed, their commonest reason for visiting emergency rooms—"but it is often overlooked by medical professionals." Though violence may occasion up to a quarter of those trips, "emergency care providers typically identify less than 5 percent of the women with injuries or illnesses suggestive of abuse."[28] And if the abusing husband or boyfriend controls an abused woman's money, insurance, or car keys, she may never get to see a doctor about her injuries at all.

A similar kind of blind spot has kept many women from getting appropriate care for another "secret" disorder, alcohol and drug abuse. Based, as we have seen, on the model of the masculine alcoholic, treatment programs may not be meeting the true needs of women. "Although not substantiated by research, the myth prevails that women have a poorer treatment prognosis than men," observes IOM's Committee for the Study of Treatment and Rehabilitation Services for Alcoholism and Alcohol Abuse.[29] Indeed, even such basic questions as whether women would benefit from a somewhat different approach, from all-female groups, or from female counselors, remain unanswered. Because substance abuse accompanies depression or other affective disorders so much more often in men than in women, the committee believes that assessing general mental health and treating depression must play a prominent role in treatment programs oriented toward females. Other useful elements, often absent from male-centered programs, include child care, support services for families, and help developing strategies for coping with stress.

"Structural barriers," in fact, seem to affect how doctors treat even so serious a condition as AIDS. When aerosolized pentamidine was the "therapy of choice," only half of all eligible patients received it. "Men were four times as likely as women" to get this optimal medication, even "after controlling for disease duration, drug use, and insurance status," noted the access committee.[30] Gay white men were likeliest of all. A similar inequity applied to use of AZT. Even "controlling for ability to pay and access to a regular source of care at a clinic," women got that cutting-edge treatment less often than gay white men. "Controlling for disease stage and past history of *Pneumocystis carinii*" as well as for "patients who received their medical care from public hospital clinics" also revealed significant bias against "minorities, women and intravenous drug users" as compared to gay white men.[31]

WHY A CRISIS IN ACCESS?

Unlike AIDS, pregnancy and childbirth are neither rare nor extremely dangerous. Unlike HIV infections, they do not call for special clinical expertise. Countless physicians know how to deliver babies; hospitals across the country own the necessary equipment and even the latest in neonatal high-tech. So why do so many expectant Americans find it impossible to get appropriate care? Why, as their due date approaches, must they undertake frantic, sometimes futile, hunts for someone to see them safely through their baby's birth?

Problems often begin with inadequate or nonexistent insurance. Mothers between 16 and 24 account for 40% of American births, but a quarter of them lack any private coverage.[32] "Once an affordable service on a middle-class income," maternity care is now, in the access committee's words, "an almost unthinkable expense without health insurance."[33] Under a third of the uninsured therefore get proper prenatal care, as opposed to 81% of the insured.[34] But neither Medicaid nor even a private policy guarantees a woman what she needs. "Because many insurance plans do not cover prenatal care and because Medicaid does not reimburse for these services at levels high enough to encourage all providers to participate, income is an important barrier to access," the access committee notes.[35] [This situation has improved in recent years, but gaps still exist (R. Gold, Alan Guttmacher Institute, personal communication, February 19, 1997).—ED.] As we have seen, a substantial proportion of American mothers receive inadequate prenatal care or essentially none at all. Such neglect helps keep "the incidence of low birthweight and of certain kinds of preventable complications of pregnancy and delivery . . . too high," observes IOM's Committee to Study Medical Professional Liability and the Delivery of Obstetrical Care.[36]

The typical American mother-to-be consults a private physician, usually an obstetrician, who also delivers the baby at a hospital. A quarter—mostly rural residents—use general practitioners or family physicians. Another 10% or so see other professionals, usually nurse-midwives.[37] But these figures mask the fact that substantial numbers of women cannot find a professional to provide continuity through the entire pregnancy and birth. They have no choice, once labor starts, but to turn up, unknown and unannounced, at whatever emergency room they can reach.

Along with inadequate health insurance, two other factors have combined to push good-quality prenatal and maternity care out of the reach of large groups and whole areas of the United States, many doctors and clinics out of the business of caring for pregnant women, and many laboring mothers into ill-prepared emergency room deliveries. The first is medical geography. Obstetrician-gynecologists, like most specialists, cluster in and around cities, leaving great stretches of countryside scantily served by the physicians best equipped to handle challenging pregnancies. Almost three dozen states have areas with fewer than 20 OB/GYNs per 100,000 women of childbearing age, almost a score have areas with fewer than 10 per 100,000, and 400,000 women in 22 states live in areas with no OB/GYNs at all.[38]

In the populous Northeast, few family doctors take obstetrical cases. In more sparsely settled regions like the North Central plains, delivering babies has long formed a routine part of general practice, and family physicians account for two-thirds of those providing private rural obstetrical care. In fact, whether a newly trained family physician wants to do obstetrics often decides if he or she begins a rural or metropolitan practice.[39]

But location goes only so far to explain the shortage of maternity services. The national crisis in malpractice liability goes the rest of the way. "Seventy percent of U.S. obstetricians can expect to be sued at one time or another," reports the liability committee. Quite apart from potential financial calamity, a lawsuit constitutes "a serious and often devastating event in the personal and professional lives" of conscientious people who work long hours and carry immense responsibilities.[40]

Both numbers of suits and the size of settlements have climbed in all medical specialties over recent decades, but most steeply in obstetrics.[41] Adding to physicians' anxiety is the knowledge that many claims brought to court may not even reflect true malpractice, in the sense of incompetent or negligent care. Desperate parents of children born with defects may have nowhere to look for help with their ruinous expenses but to the "deep pockets" of malpractice insurers. Citizens of countries with universal coverage like Britain and Canada bring many fewer such claims.

With lawsuits striking more than two out of three obstetricians, "it is abundantly clear that medical malpractice claims are not confined to the worst practitioners or the worst health care institutions," the liability committee concluded. "In fact, many observers believe that the most substandard physicians are the least likely to be sued, because they serve patients who are too poor and too uneducated to file claims. . . . Some of the best physicians are the most likely to attract suits."[42]

Medically unjustified suits, however much they may benefit certain plaintiffs, still carry a high price for other children and their mothers. "The continued increase in the frequency and severity of claims against obstetricians is compromising the delivery of obstetrical services in this country," the liability committee warns. "That effect, in turn, is reducing access to obstetrical services for certain groups of women."[43]

The ever-present possibility that any less-than-perfect outcome will precipitate an emotionally and financially draining lawsuit persuades many doctors either to refuse service to the riskiest patients or to give up obstetrics altogether. Along with the size and probability of judgments, the cost and difficulty of buying malpractice insurance have also risen rapidly. Doctors who remain in the field, whether OB/GYN specialists or family practitioners, often find that escalating insurance premiums can make delivering babies a prohibitively expensive business proposition.

Not surprisingly, these pressures hit poor patients first and hardest, both because they have more complications and low-birth-weight babies than average and because, even with Medicaid, they can cost doctors money. Some states reimburse less for a normal delivery than the physician has to pay per patient in liability premiums.[44] Staying in the obstetrics business means spending more hours on private patients who can pay their bills. The poor "end up competing with middle-class patients for the physician's time."[45] As the percentage of insured women falls, so does the doctor's ability and desire to practice this expensive specialty.

But financial cost alone is not the root of this evil. "Fear of suit may be as great a barrier to obstetrical care for low-income women as the rate of reimbursement," believes the liability committee. Refusing to accept potentially problematic cases strikes many physicians as simple prudence. "Particularly with new patients, where the likelihood of a problem pregnancy may be less clear, physicians may screen out poorer women because of their greater potential to develop high-risk pregnancies," the liability committee observes. Poor women often strike doctors as intrinsically unpromising patients, lacking the knowledge, resources, and commitment to stick to the demanding medical regimens that high-risk pregnancies may require. So how does a physician determine which low-income women to accept? "It may be easier for the physician simply to stop serving Medicaid patients entirely than to attempt to make such judgments (if desired) on an individual basis," the committee suggests.[46]

So, by default, community and migrant health centers provide much of the prenatal care that poor women do manage to obtain. But even they, in the blunt words of one center director, "are often unable to provide on-site or contract off-site prenatal care and delivery services because of the high cost of malpractice insurance."[47] For those that do treat pregnant women, paying for premiums can use up the funds needed to recruit and retain insurable OB/GYNs. Clinics may have to rely on family doctors and nurse-midwives, even though they may lack either the insurance or the credentials needed to deliver in local hospitals. Or the centers may hire newly trained obstetricians, whose lack of experience, in an actuarial absurdity, translates into lack of "accumulated exposure" to risk and thus into lower malpractice premiums.

All this leaves many centers and clinics with no choice but to turn pregnant patients away, sometimes without as much as a suggestion of where else to look for help. And those that do manage to provide prenatal care may have to abandon women as labor nears, leaving them "virtually on their own in locating delivery care."[48] Without backup or referral resources, the family physicians and nurse-midwives at these facilities find themselves "in the untenable position of having to choose whether to drop a patient at the time of delivery (and hope she could make it to the emergency room), deliver a baby without medical malpractice insurance, or cease furnishing prenatal care altogether," the liability committee observes. "Terminating care of a patient at the time of delivery not only places the patient in jeopardy and the physician into an ethical dilemma, it also creates potential liability for the physician who ultimately performs the delivery with no prior knowledge of the patient."[49]

In a cruel and dangerous irony, then, "the very factors that call for increased access to care can also intensify a physician's sense of risk when caring for low-income patients," the committee goes on. "The extent to which low-income women receive late or no prenatal care and are therefore at greater risk has been well documented. . . . Yet it is precisely this information that may underlie physicians' sense that care of low-income and Medicaid patients increases their risk of malpractice litigation."[50]

And most ironic of all, poor women actually sue no more often than their better-off sisters and win smaller judgments when they do. Poorly educated, unsure of their rights, confused by the legal system, unable to claim substantial sums in lost earnings, they often cannot find lawyers to take their cases. But these facts notwithstanding, the committee notes, "the mere perception . . . that low-income women pose professional liability problems constitutes a barrier to care."[51]

Though the liability crisis has taken its most grievous toll on the poor and minorities, its effects on obstetrics reach far up the socioeconomic ladder. Significant numbers of physicians, including OB/GYNs, have either limited the number of obstetrical cases they accept or stopped taking them altogether. Family physicians charge lower fees than obstetricians, and for many, the economics of providing obstetrical care have become particularly stark. Delivering babies substantially raises their overall liability premiums. If these cases compose only a small fraction of the total practice, the added cost of doing obstetrics can easily exceed the income it produces.

But then, "when family physicians drop obstetrics, women in rural areas are the most severely affected," the committee notes.[52] Where populations are sparse and distances great, shortages of services—even for adequately insured women—can become even more severe than among the urban poor. Scores of counties, whole regions of certain states, have no obstetrical providers. No one knows for sure how many physicians have reduced or abandoned obstetrics practice because of malpractice liability issues, but, the committee found "inescapable" "the conclusion that a sizable number are doing so."[53]

Similar liability concerns have meanwhile sharply curtailed the activities of nurse-midwives, who charge much less than physicians. Though permitted to practice in all 50 states and entitled to Medicaid reimbursement since 1980, they, too, have found insurance increasingly unobtainable. Certified nurse-midwives have a good record of safe deliveries, but nonetheless, "the difficulties in obtaining professional liability insurance in many states have made it virtually impossible for nurse-midwives to practice other than as the employees of physicians. Many nurse-midwives would prefer to form their own practices and employ physicians as consultants for high-risk or complicated deliveries. Without available insurance, however, this practice pattern, which affords maximum professional autonomy, while not illegal, is practically impossible."[54]

But even if a woman can find a doctor still doing obstetrics, she may collide with the fact that more and more now decline to take high-risk cases, regardless of the patient's coverage. Many family physicians now find it difficult to find a suitable specialist for referring or consulting about a difficult case. "Family practice obstetrics generally centers on low-risk patients," the liability committee observed. "As obstetricians reduce high-risk care, fewer referral sources are available to a rural practitioner. Furthermore, low-risk obstetrical cases can become high risk, even during delivery, and the family physician may feel particularly vulnerable to suit in such cases."[55]

CHANGING PRACTICES

Responding to these many pressures, physicians in recent decades have changed a good deal more than *whom* they treat. They have also changed *how* they treat, using more high technology and practicing more defensively. In a 1985 survey of obstetricians, for example, 41% acknowledged altering their methods because of concern about liability.[56] No matter what type of practitioner a woman sees, her maternity care probably reflects the malpractice crisis.

Of all the changes of recent decades, perhaps the most profound is the decline in the confidence and familiarity that once bound doctor and patient. In today's less personal atmosphere, as women hunt for physicians to accept them and doctors scrutinize patients as potential courtroom adversaries, "erosion of trust is both one of the causes and one of the consequences of the medical professional liability crisis," the committee believes. On the one hand, fewer and fewer Americans have long-standing family physicians whom they feel they know personally. More and more see contact with a doctor as a business relationship, and a dissatisfied client is much likelier to sue than a disappointed friend. On the other hand, the threat of litigation undermines "physicians' self-confidence and career satisfaction."[57]

These trends permeate most medical fields these days. A second change in attitude, however, uniquely affects obstetrics. Over the past several decades, notes Stephen B. Thacker, M.D., of the Centers for Disease Control and Prevention, "the obstetrician's primary concern [has shifted] from the mother to the fetus and newborn child."[58] Pressure to produce a perfect infant each and every time has increased, both as insurance claims have mounted and as highly touted new technologies have raised public expectations of medicine's ability to work wonders.

Some of the resulting changes, experts note, involve such improvements as more and better information for patients, much greater use of informed consent, and far clearer explanations of risks. But others have proven both costly and medically dubious. Consultations and referrals have increased, sometimes to benefit the patient through expert guidance, but "often," the liability committee notes, "solely for the purpose of avoiding litigation."[59] And, notes Arnold Relman, M.D., former editor-in-chief of the *New England Journal of Medicine* and professor of medicine at Harvard, "The growing—and probably excessive—use of fetal monitoring and cesarean sections undoubtedly stems in part from this fear of the legal action that might result should the pregnancy yield anything less than a perfect baby."[60]

Introduced in 1960, electronic fetal monitoring (EFM) initially appeared to offer a more reliable substitute for the century-old practice of auscultation, or listening to the fetus's heart through a stethoscope. Victorian doctors knew that an abnormally slow fetal heartbeat could spell trouble. By the end of the 1960s, EFM, including ultrasound and EKG monitoring of the fetus, was common for high-risk pregnancies. Used during labor, early observations suggested, it reduced stillbirths, injuries, and deaths. Journal articles and professional meetings extolled these advantages. By 1976, three out of four doctors surveyed believed EFM suitable for all pregnancies, and all but one of the nation's obstetrics training programs had adopted it.[61] Systematic study of EFM's efficacy, however, lagged far behind its rapid spread. Both industry and the National Institutes of Health supported development of the technology but not evaluation of its effects. Blue Cross, Medicaid, and other insurers began reimbursing without question.

Eight out of nine randomized clinical trials of EFM, however, have found little basis for the early enthusiasm. Not a single one of these studies, the liability committee reports, "has shown a statistically significant decrease in the rate of prenatal death, intraparal stillbirth . . . or frequency of neonatal intensive care admissions. . . . These studies suggest that EFM simply has not done what its proponents argued it would do: it has not reduced neonatal morbidity and death [or] the frequency of developmental disability" such as cerebral palsy.[62]

Once doctors and hospitals had invested in the equipment, though, they rapidly integrated it into both practice and teaching. Obstetricians-in-training no longer gained extensive experience with auscultation and so felt uncomfortable depending on it. The more doctors used EFM, the more patients—and especially their malpractice attorneys—came to expect it. Despite the absence of any strong evidence that it protects either mother or child, "the legal literature suggests that EFM has become the accepted standard of care in many jurisdictions," the liability committee found. "The allegation of 'failure to monitor' is commonplace in plaintiffs' medical malpractice complaints. Hospital attorneys routinely advise obstetricians both to use EFM and to save the tracing tape in case a claim is made."[63] Continuous EFM during labor has become commonplace, even for low-risk patients.

"The sole purpose of such surveillance may be only to provide a heartbeat-to-heartbeat credible objective record for defense purposes in the event of future litigation," the chairman of an obstetrics department told the liability committee. But this example, he adds, teaches new generations of physicians to de-emphasize "bedside clinical evaluation and clinical judgment" in favor of expensive technology.[64]

Did doctors in fact adopt the technique for their own rather than their patients' protection? "Although data relating EFM use to medical liability concerns are limited, it appears that the initial acceptance of EFM technology was fueled in part by such concerns," the liability committee concluded. "Moreover, the current professional liability climate supports the continued use of EFM, despite overwhelming evidence that it does not improve neonatal mortality and morbidity rates."[65]

Such self-protection might be acceptable, however, if, to paraphrase the Hippocratic Oath, it "first, did no harm." But EFM, for all its apparent lack of medical benefits, costs an estimated $750 million a year.[66] And beyond that, evidence suggests it may be in some cases actively harmful. "Although difficult to prove, it is thought that there is a higher incidence of dystocia [failure to progress in labor] among women who have continuous electronic fetal monitoring, the reason being that they are unable to walk," Thacker suggests. "They are therefore less able to tolerate labor and require more sedation."[67] In addition, the liability committee observes that "the frequency of operative deliveries, primarily cesarean sections, has been linked statistically to the use of EFM," increasing both costs and mothers' risk of injury.[68]

This rising rate of cesarean births in fact constitutes the other major change in obstetrical practice over recent decades. Certain kinds of infants who, Thacker argues, "most clinical studies have shown . . . can safely be delivered vaginally" nonetheless now routinely come into the world by cesarean. Although accepted guidelines provide for vaginally delivering such babies, "in many institutions today all infants who present by the breech are delivered by cesarean section." Thacker holds the "medi-cal-legal environment . . . responsible. With so few vaginal breech deliveries, there is less opportunity to educate residents; we have therefore an increasing pool of physicians with little or no experience in performing such deliveries."[69]

Nor do today's residents have either incentive or encouragement to learn older techniques to use in tricky situations. "For many years," the head of an obstetrics department told the liability committee, "a standard part of my teaching to medical students and residents had been to perform only medically and obstetrically indicated cesarean sections, uninfluenced by other considerations such as inconvenience, time of the day or night, interference with office hours, monetary gain, or threat of malpractice. I can no longer in good conscience continue to teach the latter principle when the practical results may be a multimillion-dollar suit that can ruin a career and a lifetime of study and service."[70]

"The high cesarean section rate in the United States is a major public health problem," Thacker warns, "one that is having and will continue to have a major impact on health care delivery. If the $800 million that could be saved by reducing the cesarean section rate by 5 percent were spent instead on prenatal care and preventive programs, dramatic effects on maternal and child health would be seen. This shift, in my opinion, is very unlikely to occur, given the current medical-legal environment, which has resulted in a siege mentality among clinicians. If one also considers that less than 20 percent on the dollar paid for malpractice premiums is given to injured parties, our current tort system is clearly very expensive, inefficient, and because of its adverse effects on the delivery of maternity care, dangerous."[71]

ELDER CARE

At the end of life, as well as at its beginning, women face specific obstacles to getting appropriate health services. They constitute the great majority of Americans who must buy long-term care—two-thirds of those needing nursing homes, 80% of those needing them for five years or more.[72] This dependence on professional caregivers represents more than women's greater longevity; it also reflects their social role.

At every age, a woman's lifetime risk of entering a nursing home is twice a man's.[73]

For all Americans, the need for long-term care rises "sharply with age, as do the effects of chronic disabling disease," notes IOM's Committee to Study the Role of Allied Health Personnel. Only 2% of those aged 65 to 74 live in nursing homes, but 32% of those above 85. But far more than age, far more than physical condition, the factor that determines who moves into an institution and who gets to stay at home is marital status. "People without spouses may not have anyone to provide the personal care that would allow them to stay in the community," the committee observes.[74] And women constitute the great bulk of elderly persons without spouses. Three-quarters of men over 65, but only a bit over one third of their female contemporaries, live in a married couple. By 85, one-third of men but only 8% of women still have a living spouse.[75]

"More women than men," Woods notes, therefore must "hire someone to provide their care."[76] Eighty-four percent of the seniors in nursing homes are not currently married, as opposed to only 64% of the similarly impaired persons able to remain outside of institutions.[77] "The typical nursing home resident is an 80-year-old white widow who has several chronic medical conditions," according to the committee. She has lived in the institution a year and a half and arrived there from a hospital. African Americans constitute only 6% of these institutionalized women, members of other races a mere 1%. Nonwhite families, the committee concludes, more often than whites care for their elderly relatives at home rather than placing them in institutions.[78]

This difference probably reflects financial exigency rather than cultural preference. Better-off people tend to have "smaller kin groups and greater financial resources," notes Barbara Silverstone, executive director of a New York social service agency, in a volume by IOM's Committee on an Aging Society. Socioeconomic status appears to explain a family's approach to long-term care better than does its race or ethnicity.[79]

One thing certain is that the cost of good-quality long-term care far exceeds most families' means. Less than half of the nation's nursing home bill was paid out of pocket in 1990, and about 40% of that from Social Security. Medicare's nursing home coverage expires after 100 days, however, with only 20 days paid in full. As a result, Medicaid pays almost half the nation's nursing home bill, but, as we have seen in other connections, sharply limits recipients' options.[80] In a pattern common among families of moderate means, the husband dies first, his final illness depleting the couple's resources. The pauperized surviving widow must then depend on public programs for her own long-term care.

Still, 42% percent of impaired elderly Americans live at home, over 80% of them dependent on family members, usually wives or adult daughters. Others hire at least some care. A study of three-generation families found that daughters in their forties and fifties averaged between 8.6 and 15 hours per week helping their aged mothers, and up to 28.5 hours if the mother lived in the daughter's home. In families that lack adult daughters, sons often pinch-hit, as do daughters-in-law.[81]

Filial devotion exacts a high price from many families. Two-thirds of those caring for an impaired elder report both physical and emotional strains. "Providing physical or nursing care" and "the elder's excessive demands for companionship" prove most burdensome, according to Silverstone. "Incontinence, immobility" and "mental abnormality" top the list of caretaker's problems, with the last the most troubling of all.[82]

Such trials eventually convince many families to place the elderly relative in a nursing home, where her welfare now depends primarily on the quality of the care provided by aides, the staff members in most frequent contact with residents. Typically a 35-year-old, high-school-educated woman who has no nursing training, an aide does a demanding job for low pay and scanty benefits. On her current job less than 2 years and in the health care field less than 5, she nonetheless carries out tasks ranging from sorting linens to observing symptoms and giving first aid. "Aides have major responsibilities for which they may have little training or experience to prepare them," the allied health committee found. "There is little status, recognition or compensation for this key role."[83] Not surprisingly, aides change jobs frequently, and nursing homes report increasing difficulty finding suitable staff. As the nation's elderly population increases, so will the demand for these key front-line workers, as well as for other allied health personnel who deal with the ailments of aging, including professionals such as physical and occupational therapists and audiologists.[84]

Exacerbating the tight market for competent aides are the

growing demands of AIDS patients. "The progression of the disease often resembles the chronic illnesses of old age (e.g., dementia and wasting)," the allied health committee writes. "AIDS patients therefore need some of the same services as the elderly and may compete for scarce resources (e.g., skilled nursing care and home health services)."[85]

But as the elderly population continues to grow, "if current morbidity, disability and functional dependence rates and patterns continue," the allied health committee predicts, "by the year 2000 about 50 percent more noninstitutionalized elderly people will require the help of others in daily living activities than required such help in 1977."[86] With more people living longer, with increasing numbers of three- and even four-generation families, and with more middle-aged women in paying jobs, the prospects for informal caregivers providing the needed help look increasingly grim. These forces may all combine to force the nation toward "a more formalized system of care," surmises IOM's Committee to Design a Strategy for Quality Review and Assurance in Medicare.[87]

Despite converging trends and hopeful forecasts, though, "the nation's stock of nursing home beds is not keeping pace with the growth in demand—let alone probable need," warns the allied health committee. "The result is that nursing homes usually have high occupancy rates and long waiting lists, thus allowing operators to select 'light' care and private-pay patients. This policy obviously works to the detriment of those who are poor and most in need of care."[88] As the number of elderly grows, that population's ratio of females to males is also rising, and since women continue to require more health services than men, those without excellent private insurance or substantial private means will find it harder and harder to get the care they need. Although older women's plight has not yet grown as desperate as that facing some of the pregnant poor, access to appropriate care promises to become even more challenging in the future.

A FEMALE GHETTO?

"In the 70s, Barbara Seaman observed that women get into the health care system via their reproductive organs," Woods says. This remains the case today. "Indeed, some would argue that women's health has become a ghetto in which only obstetricians, gynecologists, midwives, obstetrical and gynecological nurse practitioners and physician's assistants assume responsibility. Outside the women's health care ghetto, women are relatively invisible and the male is taken as the norm." Because of this distorted focus, she sees "problems in diagnosing and treating women based on assumptions that limit clinicians' ability to understand health as it is experienced by people of both genders."[89]

Because women receive much of their care from a variety of specialists focused on parts of their bodies or lives—obstetricians concerned with pregnancy, geriatricians concerned with old age—"the segmented nature of women's health services has interfered with our ability to envision health care across the life span for women," Woods continues.

So how should we organize care? Some observers argue for a new specialty in women's health, "analogous to pediatrics or geriatrics . . . oriented to a specific population rather than an organ or body system."[90] Others advocate regrouping existing specialties so that internal and family medicine form women's main source of primary care, with obstetrics and gynecology providing mainly referral for special cases and surgical services. This would entail "interdisciplinary research to address the gaps in our knowledge of how women's reproductive and endocrine cycles affect health and disease," Woods believes. In addition, "medical students would learn how to identify themselves across gender lines, all specialties would become more user friendly to women, and the medical profession would rectify its past inequities in its conceptualization of women and the denial of leadership opportunities to women. That's a tall order."[91]

But navigating today's uncoordinated and costly care system is a tall order as well, and one that women must face throughout their lives, as they try to solve their own and their families' health problems. Spurred by their unique physiological needs and often complicated by their particular social and economic situation, that challenge will grow no easier until thoroughgoing reform puts adequate health care within the reach of all Americans of both genders.

NOTES

1. IOM 1992 Annual Meeting, p. 157.
2. Ibid.
3. Ibid., 157.

4. Ibid., 156.
5. Ibid., 159.
6. Ibid.
7. Ibid., 160.
8. Ibid., 160.
9. *Toward a National Health Care Survey: A Data System for the 21st Century*, 24.
10. IOM 1992 Annual Meeting, 160.
11. Ibid., 161.
12. Ibid.
13. Ibid., 163-4.
14. Ibid., 162.
15. Ibid., 165-6.
16. *Access to Health Care in America*, 134.
17. IOM 1992 Annual Meeting, 164.
18. *Access to Health Care*, 87.
19. Ibid., 88.
20. Ibid., 87.
21. *Effectiveness and Outcomes in Health Care*, 53-4.
22. *Access to Health Care*, 89.
23. Ibid., 86.
24. Quoted ibid., 66.
25. Ibid., 85.
26. Ibid., 85-6.
27. Ibid.
28. Ibid., 134.
29. *Broadening the Base of Treatment for Alcohol Problems*, 358.
30. *Access to Health Care*, 164.
31. Ibid., 165.
32. Ibid., 27.
33. *Access to Health Care*, 41.
34. *Medical Professional Liability and the Delivery of Obstetrical Care*, Vol. II, 60.
35. *Access to Health Care*, 51.
36. Ibid.
37. Ibid., 14.
38. Ibid., 15.
39. Ibid., 18.
40. Ibid., 87.
41. Ibid., 2.
42. Ibid., 87-8.
43. Ibid., 2.
44. Ibid., 60-2.
45. Ibid., 87.
46. Ibid., 63.
47. Ibid., 69.
48. Ibid.
49. Ibid., 70.
50. Ibid., 63.
51. Ibid., 65.
52. Ibid., 47.
53. Ibid., 42.
54. Ibid., 51.

55. Ibid., 45.
56. Ibid., 75.
57. *Medical Professional Liability*, Vol. I, 87.
58. Thacker in *Medical Professional Liability*, Vol. II.
59. Ibid., 83.
60. Relman in *Medical Professional Liability*, Vol. II, 102.
61. Thacker in *Medical Professional Liability*, Vol. II, 10.
62. *Medical Professional Liability*, Vol. I, 79.
63. Ibid., 81.
64. Ibid., 83.
65. Ibid., 81.
66. Ibid., 82.
67. Thacker in *Medical Professional Liability*, Vol. II, 31.
68. *Medical Professional Liability,* Vol. I, 82.
69. Thacker in *Medical Professional Liability*, Vol. II, 23.
70. *Medical Professional Liability*, Vol. I, 83.
71. Thacker in *Medical Professional Liability*, Vol. II, 38.
72. IOM 1992 Annual Meeting, 165.
73. *Medicare: A Strategy for Quality Assurance*, Vol. I, 74.
74. *Allied Health Services: Avoiding Crises*, 261.
75. *America's Aging: Health in an Older Society*, 154.
76. IOM 1992 Annual Meeting, 165.
77. *Allied Health Services*, 262.
78. Ibid., 264.
79. Silverstone in *America's Aging*, 159.
80. IOM 1992 Annual Meeting, 165.
81. Silverstone in *America's Aging*, 158.
82. Ibid., 163.
83. *Allied Health Services*, 256.
84. Ibid., 66.
85. Ibid., 90.
86. Ibid., 261.
87. *Medicare*, Vol. I, 92.
88. *Allied Health Services*, 263.
89. IOM 1992 Annual Meeting, 166-7.
90. Ibid., 167.
91. Ibid., 168.

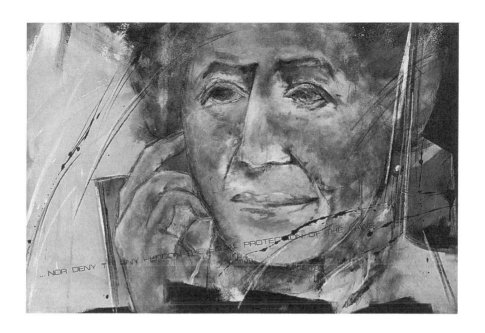

Linda Hawkin-Israel
Women in Law (1985)
Oil on canvas
The National Museum of Women in the Arts
Gift of the Foundation for Women Judges
in honor of Justice Sandra Day O'Connor

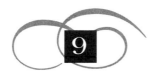

Research on Women,
Women in Research

merican biomedical research today ranks as the finest in the
world; the finest, in fact, in the history of the world. But is
this massive, prodigiously productive enterprise doing all it
can to promote women's health? For a number of years now, critics have
insisted that it does not, that several kinds of bias have kept women and
women's health issues from getting their fair share of the nation's scientific
resources. And because of this, they charge, women experience poorer
health care and thus poorer health.

The neglect, they allege, takes two main forms. Under the
guise of protecting women and children from harm, restrictive rules have
excluded reproductive-aged women—the bulk of the adult female population—from serving as subjects in clinical studies, including those investigating diseases, treatments, and medications common among women. In
addition, important health concerns like breast cancer, osteoporosis, menopause, and even pregnancy and childbirth, have gotten markedly less funding and attention than their significance in women's lives would justify.
And relatively few women belong to the ranks of scientists and
policymakers who determine research priorities.

But society has moved beyond attitudes that sanction gender-
based exclusions and inviolate medical authority. Following the lead of
AIDS activists, formerly excluded groups now assert the right to partici-

pate in trials of the latest experimental treatments. In keeping with feminist thinking, women's advocates now insist on a prominent place for female issues and investigators. Together, these demands have triggered far-reaching reexamination of who participates in research, both as subjects and as scientists.

"For the nation's research agenda to be just, it must ensure that medical research promotes the health and well-being of both men and women," states IOM's Committee on the Ethical and Legal Issues Relating to the Inclusion of Women in Clinical Studies, which was appointed to examine the policies and practices that govern who gets to participate in and who gets to perform the clinical research that provides so much of our new medical knowledge.[1] But its extensive study revealed a number of extrascientific factors that also shape research. "What many perceive to be the relative inattention to the study of health problems experienced primarily by women may arise from subtler (yet powerful) forces such as gender and race biases that permeate both society and scientific research," the committee believes.[2] In addition, the structure and funding of academic medicine have contributed to the neglect of important women's health issues.

HOW UNFAIR HAS SCIENCE BEEN?

Clinical studies—research projects that use human beings to learn about medical conditions and the effects of various treatments and interventions—provide much of the new information that helps physicians improve care. This work plays a particularly crucial role in determining which treatments work best. The normal course of a disease; the usefulness of particular diagnostic markers; the safety and efficacy of medications, surgeries, and many other kinds of treatments show up most convincingly through systematic observations of large, representative groups of people. The randomized clinical trial—a sophisticated experiment that compares the experience of one statistically valid sample of persons (randomly selected to undergo a particular treatment or intervention) with a comparable sample of persons randomly selected to be controls—is such an effective method that researchers and clinicians alike consider it the "gold standard" of proof. Treatments proven by this honored technique claim an authority that those without this backing lack.

Competing good intentions clash in the question of who should participate in these trials: science's obligation to protect experimental subjects from harm versus people's desire to gain the benefits of participating in studies. On the one hand, medicine bears the duty, as old as the Hippocratic Oath, to "first, do no harm." And, a series of medical catastrophes during the past century has impressed on researchers just how tricky that duty is to fulfill. For a variety of biological and cultural reasons, women ranked high on the list of the vulnerable victims who seemed to need protection.

But modern science, on the other hand, has also taken on the obligation to provide ever better care. And treatments can improve only to the extent that they are tested on individuals like those who will receive them in clinical practice. Even the best therapy may not work as well in persons who differ from the test population in any relevant way, be it biochemically, physiologically, genetically, or behaviorally. Thus, any group—such as women or racial minorities—that is systematically underrepresented in clinical studies runs the risk of receiving treatments tested on people unlike themselves and thus potentially less effective or even harmful.

So has biomedical research in fact slighted women? Has their health suffered as a result? Some experts answer with an unequivocal yes. "The historical lack of research focus on women's health concerns has compromised the quality of health information available to women as well as the health care they receive," found a U.S. Public Health Service task force in 1985.[3] But when the inclusion committee attempted to measure the extent of the neglect, a more complicated picture emerged. Misguided good intentions have in some cases definitely translated into inadequate medical information and resulting inferior care. But in many others, inadequate data and research design prevent any definitive answer.

Biomedical science, ironically enough, has historically paid so little attention to gender issues that even a very extensive review of the literature could not prove systematic underrepresentation of women. So few studies noted the gender of their subjects, analyzed their data by gender, or even recruited the numbers of women needed to do those analyses that accurate estimates of the full extent of women's under- (or in some cases over-) representation proved impossible. Thus, the committee could only conclude that "the available evidence is insufficient to determine whether women have participated in the whole of clinical studies to the same extent as men and whether women have been disadvantaged by policies and practices regarding their participation or a failure to focus on their health interest in the conduct of research."[4]

The committee did find two major—and life-threatening— exceptions. Though unable to "establish that gender inequity existed in the whole of past clinical research," it did find "evidence relevant to this issue in two areas of disease research: AIDS and heart disease."[5] Important research projects of these two major killers of females "either exclude women altogether or include them in numbers too small to yield meaningful information about their treatment. . . ."[6]

Coronary heart disease, "the single most frequent cause of death in women," and other heart ailments kill 500,000 American women each year and hospitalize 2.5 million. "Yet despite these compelling statistics," the committee notes, "a perception persists among the public and physicians that women do not contract heart disease as often as men and when they do, it is not as serious."[7]

Though this misconception both results from and causes gender bias, it gained credence from an impeccable research source, the highly influential Framingham project. For 12 years starting in 1948, this pioneering look at heart disease followed Massachusetts men and women aged between 36 and 68. Three times more males than females died of CHD during those years, leading researchers to the quite reasonable conclusion that middle-aged men have much greater propensity than women to death by coronary. But many also leaped to the unproved corollary that women therefore enjoy some sort of "protection" against heart disease.

Had the researchers trailed their subjects for another decade or so, a more complicated truth would have emerged: whatever "protection" women possess during their reproductive years begins to vanish with menopause. Though they rarely suffer a coronary event before age 65, their heart attack rate rises sharply by 75. "Thus, a failure to include people over 65 in clinical studies of heart disease has serious ramifications for women," the committee found, because women "develop the disease later than men and are 20 years older at their first MI [myocardial infarction—a type of heart attack]."[8]

Probably the most serious of the ramifications is that researchers, assuming they were studying a disease that mainly threatened men, concentrated their subsequent investigations of both the disease process and potential treatments almost exclusively on one gender. During the next two decades a series of influential clinical studies—the Multiple Risk Factor Intervention Trial (MRFIT), the Coronary Drug Project (CDP), the Lipid Research Clinic, and the Physicians' Health Study, used tens of thousands of men to analyze such crucial factors as the role of cholesterol and other fats in the bloodstream, the effects of fat-lowering drugs, and the potential of low-dose aspirin to prevent heart attacks. Together, these projects shaped clinical thinking as well as practice.

But by excluding women, the studies denied doctors definitive information about how to prevent, diagnose, and treat heart disease in more than half the population at risk. Extrapolating from MRFIT, CDP, and other male-based results ignores important facts about females. Estrogen, for example, may fight fatty buildup in the arteries. When heart disease does strike a woman, it often manifests itself differently from in a man. The major risk factors—high blood pressure, cigarette smoking, and obesity—hold for both genders, but certain of the familiar male early warning signs do not. In a man, coronary heart disease usually first shows up as a myocardial infarction, but in a woman as the chest pain called angina pectoris. Because women with angina may go years without an MI, many people see the female form of the disease as "less serious," even though, when an MI does finally strike a woman, she is likelier than a man to die.[9]

Do later diagnosis and less appropriate treatment contribute to that female higher death rate? No one knows for sure, but studies suggest that the treadmill test and other standard diagnostic tools developed on men may work less well on women. What's more, women receive fewer of the high-tech invasive procedures like coronary bypass surgery than equally sick men.[10] And when women do undergo that operation, they survive it less often, possibly because techniques perfected in male hearts and arteries work less well in women's smaller organs and vessels.[11]

Gender bias stands out even more starkly in AIDS. Researchers initially conceptualized the disease as an affliction of gay males, even though it appeared in women as early as 1981 and since 1986 has been rising faster in them than among men. The focus only gradually widened to include infants and male drug users. Studies that involved women much more often considered them as vectors of their babies' or their mates' infections than as victims in their own right.[12] Not until 1994 did the National Institutes of Health undertake a major project to map the disease's course and signs in women.

More typical have been studies of how women transmit the virus to sex partners or offspring. One 1990 effort tried to determine whether various methods of administering AZT could cut infection of babies during childbirth. The project's original design provided no health care for the HIV-infected mothers; a revised protocol continued the mothers' AZT for 6 weeks after birth, but the babies' for 18 months.[13] "A review of the literature yields only a handful of papers focusing on the consequences of the infection in nonpregnant women," noted a critic in 1992.[14] Questions slighted by researchers include such basic ones as how males transmit the infection to females and how women can protect themselves during sex. Much too little is known about the sexual practices that spread the virus among heterosexuals.

This blindness to women as legitimate AIDS sufferers and not simply instruments of other people's suffering has also denied them treatment opportunities available to men. The very definition of the disease developed by the Centers for Disease Control and Prevention and used to apportion disability benefits and spots in treatment programs long ignored conditions common in women. The treatments used in those programs, furthermore, had been tested for effectiveness on men rather than women. Nearly all studies of how people cope with the disease have concentrated on gay men. "Finally," notes the inclusion committee, "in clinical trials of AIDS drugs, which often may provide significant sources of first-rate medical care and access to experimental treatments for persons with AIDS, the numbers of women participating lags behind expectations for a disease that is increasing the most rapidly among women."[15]

Another life-threatening area where research lags is women's addictions. "The classical studies that have informed our thinking about alcohol," Blume observes, such as "George Vallian's wonderful book, *The Natural History of Alcoholism*, Chuck Snyder's very interesting book, *Alcohol and the Jews*, should really be entitled *Natural History of Alcoholism in Men* and *Alcohol and Jewish Men*, because neither study contained a single subject that was female."[16] The course of the disease in women remains unclear, as does its specifically feminine relationship to depression. Only recently have screening instruments suitable for women become available, although none exists yet that adequately deals with teenage girls.

Sometimes missing knowledge means great danger. "There have been many studies of the techniques of detoxification from alcohol, books full. There is none that I could find on the best way to detoxify a pregnant woman," Blume laments. "Of all the phone calls I get from psychiatrists and other physicians around the country, that is the most common question."[17] Pregnancy is only the most dramatic of the special situations about which researchers know very little. Almost no research exists on the issues that alcoholism raises in women prisoners, students, HIV patients, and seniors, or among lesbians or minority women. "We know that sociocultural factors are important in shaping the development of women's alcohol problems, but we know nothing about how to apply these factors to case finding, to treatment."[18]

HOW HAS SCIENCE BEEN UNFAIR?

Treating women unfairly shortchanges their health in two major ways. First and most obviously, science knows less than it could about both conditions that affect only women and how the two genders experience conditions that affect them both. Does a given disease act identically? Do the different physiologies and biochemistries of males and females—and of females at various stages of the life course—affect diagnosis or response to treatment? Is a drug, surgery, or other treatment proven useful for one gender equally suitable for the other? If studies do not include adequate numbers of both men and women, these questions go unanswered—and usually even unasked.

But asking these questions each and every time is not necessary, many experts believe. Both researchers and clinicians generally assume that drugs effective on one group of people will work equally well in others, barring a compelling biological reason to the contrary.[19] "Basically, the question can be rephrased, 'Will differences in drug disposition or drug response due to gender be clinically significant?' " writes Leslie Z. Benet, Ph.D., chairman of the Department of Pharmacy at the University of California, San Francisco. "My answer is, 'Rarely, if ever.' "[20]

Most drugs available today, Benet notes, have a wide enough margin between a therapeutic dose—the amount or blood concentration needed for a beneficial effect—and the toxic dose—the amount that is poisonous—to accommodate quite a wide range of individual differences. The effects of drugs with narrower margins (known technically as the therapeutic index) between potency and peril tend to vary considerably among individuals, so doctors find the right dose by titrating them individually for each patient. "It is my hypothesis," Benet argues, "that the health consequences of the exclusion or underrepresentation of women in clinical studies for narrow therapeutic index drugs will be minimal, since it is immaterial whether women differ significantly from men . . . since in each case the drug will be titrated by the clinician to the appropriate dose or concentration." And even in wide therapeutic index drugs, "there should be few health consequences for large gender differences . . . since the variability inherent in the male population most likely already encompasses the difference between the male and female populations."[21]

Still, the "known biological, behavioral and social differences between the genders . . . are real and significant," the inclusion committee insists, and "can affect response to drugs and other treatments, creating the potential for differential health consequences. . . ."[22] Benet himself favors including women in trials, because of differences like the recently discovered variation in drug metabolism between pre- and postmenopausal women.

And male-oriented medicine does cause problems in areas other than heart disease, addiction, and AIDS. Women seem to suffer more adverse drug reactions.[23] Even in apparently well-understood conditions, physicians may hesitate to give females drugs or treatments proven safe only in males, depriving them of some of the newest advances.[24] More strikingly still, enormously common female conditions like fibroid tumors and preeclampsia of pregnancy remain poorly understood. Women even lack clear medical guidance for dealing with the universal and normal hormonal changes of menopause. "When it comes to health problems like these involving obstetrics and gynecology, our lack of knowledge is enormous," writes Mary Lake Polan, M.D., chair of obstetrics and gynecology at Stanford University Medical School and member of an IOM committee studying research efforts in academic OB/GYN departments. "Why are babies born prematurely? Why have ectopic pregnancies, those outside the uterus, increased every year since 1970, with a fatality rate of 42 per 1,000 cases? Why hasn't our understanding of sexually transmitted diseases like herpes, genital warts and AIDS kept up with the sexual revolution? Why? Because our effort to find answers has been half-hearted and inadequate."[25]

WHY EXCLUSION?

In keeping women out of the great majority of clinical studies, scientific policymakers intended to do good rather than harm, to decrease rather than increase the sum of human suffering, to protect a vulnerable population—or, more accurately, two vulnerable populations—from what they perceived as great but unknown dangers. Although some clinical research involves nothing more dangerous than comparing the medical records of different groups, much of it entails experiments that may pose unknown hazards.

And this century has a sordid history of human experimentation. "Public outcry and tragedy have driven policy development in the area of research on human subjects," note ethicist Tracy Johnson, M.A., of the Bass & Howes consulting firm and historian Elizabeth Fee, Ph.D., professor of history and health policy at Johns Hopkins School of Hygiene and Public Health.[26] In 1938, after a drug called Elixir Sulfanilamide killed 107 people, Congress required, in the Food, Drug and Cosmetics Act of 1938, that manufacturers prove medications safe before bringing them to market. That meant they had to test them on humans. Under the previous Food and Drug Act, passed in 1906, proof of strength and purity had been the only requirements.

But human experimentation gained a particularly gruesome reputation in the 1940s when the Nuremberg war crimes trials revealed to a horrified world the extent of atrocities committed by Nazi doctors on helpless prisoners in the name of medical science. Growing out of world-wide revulsion at this officially sanctioned savagery, the Nuremberg Code guaranteed to every person acting as a research subject the right of free and fully informed consent to any risks entailed in any study. The code further stipulated that subjects must possess the capacity to give that consent, that human experimentation must take place only when potential benefits outweigh risks, and that there must be no other possible method to obtain the desired information.

But these provisions did not end exploitation of the vulnerable. In the 1960s and 1970s a shocked American public learned of abuses that bore disturbing parallels to wartime excesses. In 1963 an experiment using live cancer cells on unwitting elderly patients came to light at the Jewish Chronic Diseases Hospital in Brooklyn, New York. Two years later, the Harvard anesthesiologist Henry K. Beecher gained national attention with a speech and subsequent paper in the *New England Journal of Medicine* describing published studies that did not fulfill the ethical requirement that subjects understand risks. "It must be apparent," Beecher wrote, "that they would not have been available if they had been truly aware of the uses that would be made of them."[27] Next, with racist overtones reminiscent of the Nazi period, came revelations about the Tuskeegee Syphilis Study. This infamous government-funded project had since 1932 observed the disease's course in a group of some 400 African American men. Although antibiotics had become the widely available, well-established treatment for syphilis midway through the project, researchers had failed to treat some of these impoverished, uneducated men or even to inform them of the possibility of treatment.

Public outrage led to a number of legislative and regulatory reforms tightening procedures and protections for experimental subjects in general. Two other traumatic episodes soon focused attention on the risks to women (and their babies) in particular. Though the tragedies involving thalidomide and DES did not involve research subjects, they drastically heightened fears of drug effects during pregnancy. Together they alerted scientists and terrified the public about the perils of exposing pregnant or even potentially pregnant women to unproved drugs.

Both disasters involved freely available medications whose effects during pregnancy, as events tragically revealed, had not been sufficiently tested. In both cases, in fact, early signs of impending trouble had been ignored. In the early 1960s the birth of nearly 8,000 severely deformed infants, born mainly in Europe, riveted the world's attention on thalidomide, an over-the-counter sleeping tablet their mothers had taken while pregnant. Though sold in 20 countries, it failed to receive FDA clearance for sale in the United States because of a regulator's suspicions about early results. Still, although this country missed the disaster's main brunt, some "investigating" doctors got it from the manufacturer and distributed it here. Despite the small number of cases on this side of the Atlantic, Americans, like people around the world, experienced "a powerful emotional impact that created an aversion to involving pregnant women and women of childbearing age in drug research," the inclusion committee notes.[28]

Then, as if to underline the point, a second drug-related disaster, this time involving large numbers of American families, came to light less than a decade later. The artificial hormone DES, widely prescribed during the 1940s and 1950s to prevent miscarriage, did less visible but still grievous damage. A rare form of vaginal cancer began appearing in "DES daughters"—girls exposed to the drug in utero—as they reached young womanhood.

Neither of these calamities resulted, as Johnson and Fee point out, from dangerous research on expectant mothers. The blame lay on "*inadequate* testing and *ignored* research results which indicated the potential for reproductive harm in women." Logically, then, these cases would seem to argue for more, rather than less, research into drug effects in pregnancy, provided it could be conducted with a stringent regard for safety.

In the ensuing uproar, though, a "counterintuitive" result won out: strong discouragement for future inclusion of anyone who was, or conceivably could become, pregnant. Ironically, though, because a certain number of pregnant women will always need medical treatment, this protective approach prevents gathering the very information needed to forestall future drug disasters. "Presumably, an all-male study population would not have shielded the manufacturers of thalidomide from liability claims of a drug marketed to women," Johnson and Fee observe.[29]

The net result of these calamities was a tightening of regulations and policies governing participation in research studies, especially by women of "reproductive potential." The FDA recommended that, except in the case of life-threatening illnesses, no one in that category take part in any early-stage drug trials, which pose the greatest risks of toxicity, regardless of her current marital status, condition of pregnancy or nonpregnancy, state of fertility, future childbearing plans, or personal desires. That policy also discouraged women's exclusion from the later-stage testing needed to determine effectiveness and appropriate dosage. And beyond official requirements, drug companies established exclusionary policies of their own. Stunned by the huge liabilities of previous disasters involving pregnant women, they eschewed research subjects who could expose them to any similar catastrophe in the future.

TOWARD INCLUSION

During the very years that the exclusionary consensus was building, however, almost unnoticed amongst the advancing restrictions, a small movement of dissenters took its first tentative steps. The DES revelations coincided with the upsurge of the modern feminist movement. Small groups of activist women began to work for greater control over their own health and health care. Such early advocacy groups as the Boston Women's Health Collective and the National Women's Health Network started to challenge the assumptions underlying a health care system they saw as paternalistic and unsympathetic to women's concerns. In 1973 the Boston group's book *Our Bodies, Ourselves* brought this view to a nationwide readership.

Feminist health activists saw the issues behind scandals over DES and the Dalkon Shield as involving (because of reports that, for example, women were given DES without their knowledge), in Johnson and Fee's words, "inappropriate *inclusion* (rather than exclusion)."[30] Rejecting the general panic, they called for more rather than less research into the common but understudied conditions that affect women. Rather than the moratorium on new knowledge that protectionist exclusion implied, they sought both more research and greater protections for those who would participate.

But the main drive to overturn the nation's protectionist policies came not from women but from men, specifically, the male homosexuals responding to the dearth of effective treatments for AIDS. Like all drugs under FDA supervision, unproved AIDS treatments were subject to strict safety rules that kept them out of the hands of most patients and many out of this country altogether. From the early years of the epidemic, activists denounced as a cumbersome, deadly waste of time the very drug approval system established by public demand to ensure safety in the wake of past abuses. Like the proverbial general fighting the last war, FDA used a strategy designed to prevent another thalidomide disaster. It only permitted drugs to come to market after a long testing process intended to protect subjects and the public from all possible risks.

AIDS activists, however, had no interest in being protected. They represented not healthy people seeking to avoid unnecessary injury but desperately ill people seeking relief from an incurable and inexorably fatal disease. They wanted to try new drugs, and they wanted them fast, so they willingly tolerated risks unacceptable to ordinary people. Through the lens of their disease, doomed victims saw experimental drugs not as unknown perils but as potentially lifesaving opportunities, and established procedures not as necessary prudence but as needless impediments. AIDS patients' only hope, they argued, lay in unproved but promising treatments inching their way through the FDA's obstacle course. Without access to these possibly lifesaving substances, sufferers faced an inevitable doom. In these desperate new circumstances, the AIDS movement insisted, old safeguards were less than useless; they were positively harmful.

In rejecting protectionism for its own sake, the AIDS activists echoed a watershed document that had appeared several years before the epidemic entered scientific consciousness. "Beneficence . . . requires that . . . we be concerned about the loss of substantial benefits that might be gained from research," stated the National Commission for the Protection of Human Subjects of Biomedical and Behavioral Research in its 1978 Belmont Report.[31] Protection was necessary, the report acknowledged, but the true purpose of research is progress that can lessen suffering. To balance risk against benefit, the report enumerated three ethical principles. The first, respect for persons, recognized the right of individuals to be treated as autonomous agents capable of making their own decisions, unless some specific factor diminishes that autonomy and necessitates protection. The second principle, beneficence, entails the obligation to seek maximum benefit and minimum harm. Finally, the principle of justice requires that risks and benefits be fairly distributed among the groups composing the population. That means that women as well as men should participate.

In 1987, after more than half a decade of further discussion and dispute, the FDA incorporated these three principles and the AIDS community's concerns into a new research policy, making experimental treatments for severe or fatal conditions available to properly informed patients earlier in the approval process, before final testing was complete. The specific issues involving women's participation, however, took several more years to come to a head.

On the scientific front, the change came slowly. As early as 1981, for example, as the first AIDS cases were coming to scientific attention, a little-noticed article in the journal *Annals of Internal Medicine* had shown that excluding reproductive-aged women from Phase I drug trials tended to keep them out of Phase III trials as well. "That the article stirred so little response reflects the relative consensus at the time among researchers and federal policy makers vis-à-vis protectionist policies governing research on women," Johnson and Fee observe.[32] This consensus gradually began to shift, however, and in 1986 the National Institutes of Health introduced a policy of encouraging more use of women as research subjects, but made little progress toward implementation.

Demography finally forced the issue. By the late 1980s the huge baby boom generation was moving into midlife. This largest, best-educated, and most professionally successful cohort of women in the nation's history had entered the age bracket that brings the first signs of aging, including menopause and rising incidence of breast and other reproductive cancers. Now this gigantic, highly self-aware age group, which since babyhood had wrenched the nation's attention to whatever issues it was currently facing, began coming to grips with how much science had yet to learn about female aging. Their dawning awareness, combined with the general growth of health advocacy in the wake of AIDS, changed women's place in research from a bureaucratic footnote to a major political issue.

Uproar rather than indifference greeted a 1990 General Accounting Office report detailing NIH's slow pace toward reform. In the light of women's new role and consciousness, "practices and policies once presented as protective were now labeled as paternalistic and discrimina-tory," the inclusion committee observes. "The rationales behind a num-ber of clinical studies that had proceeded without question were now being questioned. Why had the NIH-sponsored Multiple Risk-Factor Intervention Trials of heart disease not included women when women as well as men were dying of heart disease? How could the Baltimore Longi-tudinal Study of Aging include no women when the elderly population in this country is disproportionately female?"[33]

In September 1990, responding to rising public and congres-sional pressure, NIH established the Office of Research on Women's Health. From its place within the office of the director of the nation's premier biomedical research funding agency, ORWH would work, ac-cording to an NIH document "1. to strengthen and enhance research related to diseases, disorders and conditions that affect women and to ensure that research conducted and supported by NIH adequately ad-dresses issues regarding women's health; 2. to insure that women are appropriately represented in biomedical and behavioral research studies supported by NIH; and 3. to foster the increased enrollment of women in biomedical research—especially in pivotal decisionmaking roles within clinical medicine and the research environment."[34] The NIH Revitaliza-tion Act of 1993 made ORWH a permanent entity and called for in-creased research funding for reproductive cancers, osteoporosis, contra-ception, and fertility. Though vetoed by President Bush in June 1992 over the issue of fetal tissue research, it was reintroduced, passed, and signed by President Clinton, who opposed the ban on fetal research, in 1993.

In 1991, meanwhile, new directives from NIH and the Alco-hol, Drug Abuse and Mental Health Administration, the major federal funder of psychological and behavioral research, required representation of women and racial minorities in clinical studies. Now, instead of having to justify *including* women on the basis of the seriousness of the condition under study, researchers had to justify *excluding* them.

Later that same year, Bernadine Healy, M.D., NIH's first fe-male director, announced the largest study of women's health ever under-taken. The $625 million Women's Health Initiative would, in fact, be the largest study that NIH had ever funded, period. Plans called for WHI to enlist numerous research centers to run a major clinical trial, as well as an observational study and community intervention projects. So costly and complex an undertaking naturally attracted much comment and criticism. As controversy grew, NIH, at the behest of the Appropriations Committee of the U.S. House of Representatives, contracted with IOM to assess the proposal's scientific merit and feasibility. The study committee suggested several modifications of the original research design, but still concluded that "valuable scientific information could be obtained in the redesigned study," although "much of the information could be obtained in better designed, smaller, more focused studies that could have a greater chance of success and probably be less costly."[35] In short, the committee gave its go-ahead for a modified WHI.

Important aspects of that decision, however, lay, in the WHI committee's words, "beyond science," in the realm of politics and public opinion.[36] Try though it might to limit its deliberations to technical issues like cost and methodology, "the committee was constantly faced with broader considerations. Colleagues, advocacy organizations, executive and legislative branch representatives, all approached the committee with reasons why the WHI should proceed, and why canceling it would unleash disasters. If canceled, some argued, no one would ever trust the government again; it would prove that the government does not really care about women's health; it would so greatly disappoint the community which has gathered around this project that it will be impossible ever to galvanize them again; it would be seen as an unwelcome political blow to those who have pressed for more women's health research. Others argued that it would be wrong and harmful to women's health to spend $625 million and find after 14 years that little in the way of useful information had been learned. It would not help women's health and women's health research to publicly announce and then misuse an enormous amount of money."[37]

Struggling to consider only "the merits of the science," the committee called the side issues "important" but declined to comment on them further. "With the committee recommendation that the WHI could proceed—though with significant changes of duration and focus—the discussion of these issues should continue," it suggested[38] And even more importantly, "whatever the merits of WHI, the committee has no doubt about the need for a substantial investment in research on women's health."[39]

MAKING INCLUSION WORK

But political pressure and increased funding alone will not succeed in reorienting research to better serve women's needs. Only a change in the culture surrounding science can fully accomplish that. "As in all scientific endeavors," notes the inclusion committee, "clinical studies seek to achieve results that are unbiased by the preconceptions of preferences of investigators, staff or study participants. This does not mean that the conduct of science is necessarily objective."[40]

Like all human beings, scientists see their experience—including their professional work—through "lenses" provided by their culture. "Basic, hidden assumptions involving gender—so basic as to be transparent—are 'lenses' through which people perceive, conceive and discuss social and scientific reality," the committee believes. Ancient notions about gender differences and social roles still strongly distort Americans' perceptions. "It is important to look *at* those lenses in order to understand their consequences, instead of looking *through* them."[41]

"Two types of gender-based assumptions" shape the vision of biomedical scientists, the committee notes.[42] "*Male bias* refers to the 'observer bias' present in scientific inquiry when scientist-observers adopt male perspectives. *Male norm* refers to the tendency to perceive men's identity and experience as the characterization or standard of what it is to be a person and to portray female differences, where they occur, as 'deviant.' "[43]

These influences shape both the questions that scientists consider important enough to investigate and the conclusions that they reach about them. In the nineteenth century, when female higher education was a controversial innovation, perfectly reputable investigators argued that studying could, by drawing energy from the uterus to the brain, damage fertility. Educated women, they observed, bore relatively few children. As ludicrous as this theory now seems, the same tendency persists to view women in terms of their social and reproductive roles rather than as complete individuals in their own right. "Historically," note

Johnson and Fee, "medical and public health professionals have conflated women's health with reproductive and child health"[44]—a propensity most chillingly illustrated in the AIDS work.

Indeed, the very subject matter of certain specialties, domains of knowledge supposedly determined by logical criteria, may reflect masculine outlooks. "The fields of sports medicine, psychiatry and occupational medicine would focus on different issues if women's recreational and nonrecreational activities and stresses dominated," the committee suggests. "Indeed, the specialties themselves might have developed differently, focusing on leisure activities instead of 'sports,' or on the hazards of domestic activities instead of the workplace."[45]

Had women's rather than men's concerns prevailed, questions that engage gynecological researchers might also have evolved differently. Study might have concentrated on such common, debilitating, and inadequately understood problems as preeclampsia, which complicates pregnancies and damages babies, or fibroid tumors, "the major cause of hysterectomies in this country," according to Polan.[46] Instead, the "substantial body of research directed at gaining control over women's reproduction" has followed a male-oriented agenda, suggests Susan Sherwin, Ph.D., professor of philosophy at Dalhousie University in Canada.

Only in this area have women received a disproportionately large share of research attention. "For example, almost all contraceptive research has explored means of controlling women's fertility. Similarly, efforts to relieve infertility have focused on procedures that can be done to women—even when the infertility is associated with such male conditions as low sperm count. As a result, a disproportionate share of the burden, risks, expenses and responsibility for managing fertility now belongs to women, because that is where the knowledge base is. . . . The concentration of attention on women's reproductive role not only assumes the conventional view that women are, by nature, to be responsible and available for reproductive activities; it also legitimizes, reinforces, and further entrenches such views and the attitudes that accompany them."[47] Even in the "science of women," therefore, as in all other medical specialties and in the training of medical personnel, the male norm has historically held sway.

Many clinical researchers, seeking to keep research designs as

simple as possible, prefer not to take account of monthly hormonal fluctuations—in other words, to study men. "One of the reasons that women
have traditionally been excluded from clinical studies of conditions that
affect both men and women is, as *The Washington Post* put it, 'their hormonal fluctuations [have been] said to "confound" or confuse research
results,' " reports Debra DeBruin, Ph.D., assistant professor of psychology
at the University of Pittsburgh. "Women's cycles appear not only to be
different from men's physiology, but also to be problematic. Because men
are conceived of in gender-neutral terms as paradigmatic persons, researchers too often feel they can simply avoid the 'problems' caused by
women's cycles by studying only men."[48]

The preference for males shows up especially strongly in drug
studies because, in the committee's words, "women have menstrual cycles
that produce deviations from the 'normal' pattern of drug disposition
observable in males."[49] But what appears a mere "confounder" in the
laboratory becomes a potential danger in the consulting room. Women
older than 60 use half of all cholesterol-lowering medications prescribed
in this country, but three-quarters of the clinical trials testing those drugs
enrolled only middle-aged men. The "deviations" that complicate researchers' statistical tables thus may produce real complications on the
examining table. Doctors therefore face two unsatisfactory alternatives:
they can either decline to prescribe for women treatments tested only in
men or assume that existing test results apply to everyone. The first deprives half the population of potentially useful therapies, but the latter
exposes them to potential risks.

Demographic "deviations" also keep women out of clinical
studies. Organizers of the Physician's Health Study, for example, found
that 90% of the appropriately aged medicos were male; the profession
included too few middle-aged females to provide the desired statistical
power. "The investigators' reservations regarding the ability to perform
such an analysis were sound," the committee found, but a more imagina-
tive approach to including women could have produced useful results.
"The enrollment of a specified subgroup does not obligate [investigators]
to perform interaction analysis for that subgroup, nor does the analysis
need to be definitive if performed. If nothing else, the size and sign of any
differences observed for women would have provided some general indi-

cation of whether the result obtained in men is consistent with that observed in, and thus generalizable to, women."[50] Had these researchers wanted to learn about women, in other words, they could have settled for a less-than-perfect but still potentially enlightening project. Indeed, the Boston Nurses Study, a large longitudinal project, is now focusing on women's health concerns.

FINDING A BALANCE

Like all human undertakings, the new policy of encouraging use of both genders in all studies has the vices of its virtues. To ensure statistical power, numbers of subjects will need to be larger and studies more expensive. "Scientific considerations suggest that the overarching principle should be inclusion," the inclusion committee believes.[51] But in an era of tight budgets, the need to stretch scarce research funds, to get the most data for each dollar, has become a principle almost as elevated. MRFIT, for example, excluded women precisely for budgetary reasons. Finding the 12,866 men who ultimately participated meant interviewing, taking blood pressure, and doing blood workups on almost 362,000 individuals. "Including women might have produced valuable information," the committee suggests, "but at a substantial additional cost."[52]

Substantially raising studies' costs, no matter how noble the motive, might significantly reduce their number, which would also mean less knowledge. "The committee is concerned that the policy has gone too far by insisting that each and every clinical trial be designed to ensure sufficient numbers of subjects of both genders to permit subgroup analyses. In an era of concern about the nation's resources, and about expenditures on health in particular, we argue that a trial-by-trial application of this requirement is neither good policy nor good science. Clinical trials should include both genders, but requiring scientists to enroll sufficient numbers to ensure the statistical power to detect unsuspected and implausible gender differences would produce little additional information at greatly increased cost."[53]

Instead of raising the cost and complexity of each and every study, "mechanisms are needed at the national level to ensure that more attention is paid to questions of justice and gender in the setting of research agendas, and at the study level to encourage the appropriate consideration of gender-related effects in clinical studies."[54] Few changes could bring about those results more quickly, many believe, than a sharp increase in the number of women entering scientific careers and advancing to leadership.

THE SCIENCE OF WOMAN

An obvious place to look for female research leadership is the nation's departments of obstetrics and gynecology, where women already account for the majority of residents and junior faculty members. Only pediatrics, public health, and physical medicine claim more female faculty.[55] Currently heavily concentrated at the lower academic ranks, this new generation ought to gain increasing power in the years ahead, as they rise to the more senior positions that influence policy in both their own hospitals and medical schools and the specialty at large. Ironically, though, this trend may actually reduce the amount of research conducted in OB/GYN departments.

Though the specialty deals with some of the central issues and experiences that women face throughout their lives, it has traditionally placed a low priority on research. At a time when science is racing toward solutions to some of the most fundamental mysteries of life itself, very basic (and probably less complicated) gynecologic questions remain unanswered: How do the ovaries, uterus, and other reproductive organs function? How does fertilization happen? What factors affect fetal development? What determines when labor begins? How can delivery be safer? What will afford safer and more effective contraception and infertility treatments? How can sexually transmitted diseases and reproductive cancers best be controlled? What is the best way to deal with menopause and premenstrual syndrome?

This ignorance translates daily into potentially preventable suffering and death. Such "large-scale problems" as the 7% of all babies born at perilously low weights; the 2.6% of all pregnancies dangerously complicated by high blood pressure; the rising numbers of ectopic pregnancies, fatal in over 4% of cases; the 10% of married couples who want children but cannot conceive; and the scores of millions of sexually transmitted infections all "could be ameliorated" by more research, believes IOM's Committee on Research Capabilities of Academic Departments of Obstetrics and Gynecology.[56] So could our nation's serious dearth of effective contraceptive options.

Despite these obvious needs, the heads of OB/GYN departments confided to the committee that financial realities make it "particularly difficult to conduct research."[57] Earning the scientific credentials needed to win research funding in today's extremely competitive environment can add several more meagerly paid fellowship years to the specialty and subspecialty training that already stretches for as much as eight years beyond medical school. And new OB/GYNs emerge from that training with both very large debts and the potential for very high incomes practicing one of the most lucrative of all specialties. Medical school departments thus must often offer a great deal—as much as $150,000 a year, according to some reports—to entice promising newcomers to choose academics over private practice. To pay these salaries at the same time that they absorb the high costs of malpractice insurance and the many uninsured women who deliver in teaching hospitals, OB/GYN departments need large incomes from paying patients. Earning them forces faculty to concentrate heavily on clinical care, "often at the expense of investigation."[58]

Lack of time and research focus thus creates a vicious circle. If a department cannot afford to support topflight laboratories, it cannot create the environment to nurture young scientists through the long process of training and mentoring that leads to productive research careers. Without young talent entering a department, it never develops the "critical mass" of ability, commitment, stimulation, and opportunity that marks a major research center. Without such a reputation, it is less able to garner research funds. This leaves it no choice but to pay its bills through patient care, depriving the faculty of time for the laboratory.

"The ethos of a discipline determines its direction," the committee believes, and much of OB/GYN has traditionally lacked leaders convinced that "research within the discipline is a high priority." Only a dozen or fewer departments "can be counted as serious research centers"; almost two score receive no federal research funding at all.[59] These facts add up to "cause for concern about the current and future state" of OB/

GYN research. "It is important to expand the number of departments that can succeed in the competitive research arena," the committee believes.[60] Bolstering the supply of physician-researchers is crucial to that goal.

One might expect that the recent, overwhelming influx of women into the field should help turn things around. Unlike their male colleagues, female doctors do not generally weigh income heavily in choosing a specialty or career direction.[61] Many also feel a strong commitment to improving women's health. But females have traditionally tended much less often than males to become researchers, a fact "likely to increase the shortage of research personnel unless special efforts are made to encourage research careers for women and to meet their particular needs."[62]

And those needs are substantial, because women face "special obstacles in choosing the laboratory over clinical practice," Polan notes. The dilemmas of joining the rigid race for tenure with one's "biological clock" ticking in the background, of doing the grueling work that leads to a secure academic position while raising small children, and of finding one's way in a male-dominated research culture all discourage would-be investigators. "Providing mentors, flexible work arrangements or extended time to gain tenure all could ease these pressures," she suggests.[63] As departments become increasingly aware of these issues, they have begun taking steps to resolve them.

The currently missing cadre of committed and talented young researchers, however, only partially explains one of the central paradoxes of American reproductive medicine. Why has the nation that once led the world in the development of safe and effective contraceptives essentially abandoned the quest for new solutions to today's ever more pressing needs? Why has the scientific community that brought the world into the age of discretionary parenthood produced no significant advances since the breakthrough developments of the 1960s? Like Sherlock Holmes's famous dog who did nothing in the nighttime, American contraceptive research has been conspicuous for its silence for over a generation.

At least since the 1980s, fewer and fewer young investigators have entered this endeavor. The "undesirable thinness in the field" that this has produced leads in turn to a "sparse literature" on new research, warns IOM's Committee on Population.[64] Clinical studies of new methods often fail to get the replicating studies they need to establish sound data on effectiveness, for example. But able new scientists do not ignore or abandon a once-promising field for no reason. A combination of factors, prominent among them that old nemesis of medical flexibility, the liability crisis, has systematically removed the incentives for aggressive contraceptive research and development in this country.

In the 1960s heyday of birth control studies, nine major U.S. pharmaceutical companies—such giants as Syntex; Searle; Parke-Davis; Merck, Sharpe & Dohme; Upjohn; Mead Johnson; Wyeth-Ayerst; and Eli Lilly—all maintained active programs in what appeared a fast-moving field. In addition, other companies like A.H. Robins, which produced the infamous Dalkon Shield, also brought products to market. Corporations annually invested millions of dollars in costly, long-term research and development programs aimed at meeting the huge demand for modern contraceptives. Private sources also contributed handsomely; the Committee on Research in Problems of Sex, for example, bankrolled by the Rockefeller family, supported work that led to the Pill. Starting in the 1960s, substantial federal funds also went toward birth control efforts.

By the 1990s, only Ortho Pharmaceutical, a Johnson & Johnson subsidiary, continued the corporate effort. Government funding had fallen as well. In place of millions of annual corporate, philanthropic, and federal dollars, total spending had dropped sharply. Young, and even middle-aged, scientists seeking career opportunities were looking elsewhere. Lack of neither promising research leads toward potential male and female contraceptives nor potentially eager customers drove these firms from the field, however. Rather, it became increasingly difficult to make a profit by getting expensive-to-develop new products into the hands of buyers.

The Dalkon Shield disaster hit contraceptive research like an atomic bomb, leveling much of the corporate landscape and contaminating what remained with long-lasting legal and regulatory fallout. Liability insurance, already becoming increasingly difficult to obtain, rose drastically in cost in the wake of the billions of dollars of claims against Robins' defective product. Companies found it increasingly difficult to justify the expensive, multiyear projects needed to develop and test new contraceptives, given the unpredictability of scientific success and regulatory approval. Firms began withdrawing from sale effective intrauterine devices that had none of the faults of the Dalkon Shield, simply because profitably defending lawsuits appeared impossible. Today, the shrunken research field consists primarily of small firms that often lack the resources for major undertakings and of projects supported by nonprofit organizations.

In other countries with other regulatory and insurance arrangements, progress has continued apace, however. In the United States, manufacturers must present convincing evidence that contraceptives are safe before they can obtain FDA approval. In Britain, on the other hand, products can win approval if the evidence shows that they are not unsafe. This disparity permitted Depo-Provera on the contraceptive market in the United Kingdom but not, based on examination of identical data, in this country. "The difference in outcome seems to have resulted not from scientific differences, but from policy differences (burden of proof) in the two countries," the population committee concluded.[65]

The United States cannot begin to meet its people's contraceptive needs unless the climate becomes considerably more hospitable, the committee believes. Although manufacturers must satisfy the FDA's stringent safety standards, for example, they cannot rely on that official approval as legal proof of safety or even of a sincere attempt to provide safety. Such rules "can be changed to remove most of their undue negative consequences" without "increasing the health risks of contraceptive users," the committee believes.[66] It suggests that the same should happen to the balance of risks and benefits currently used to judge contraceptives. Because an unwanted pregnancy can impose serious health risks on some women, "methods with fewer side effects are not necessarily safer if they have higher failure rates." The committee, however, "does not propose reducing the safety requirements," but rather "adding new criteria" to make safety evaluations "more specific to different groups of users."[67]

Despite the various "obstacles" standing in the way of better reproductive health, however, the obstetrics committee nonetheless sees "several encouraging signs," including an increase in programs to support OB/GYN researchers and a growing engagement among the field's leadership in the need to encourage research. For all their problems, though, these trends, coupled with the general drive to include more women in research, both as subjects and as investigators, hold promise of greater knowledge and better health for women in years to come. Indeed, because of "increasing interest in women's health issues," the committee believes, "the 1990s offer an unprecedented opportunity" for progress.[68] As long-hidden biases come to light and outmoded restrictions fall away, American biomedical research can increasingly become not only the world's most productive, but also among the world's most just.

NOTES

1. *Women and Health Research: Ethical and Legal Issues of Including Women in Clinical Trials*, Vol. 1, 28.

2. Ibid., p. 37.

3. Quoted in *Women and Health Research*, Vol. 1, 43.

4. *Women and Health Research*, Vol. 1, 49.

5. Ibid.

6. Ibid.

7. Ibid, 64.

8. Ibid.

9. Ibid, 65.

10. Weisman and Cassard, *Women and Health Research*, Vol. 2, 37.

11. Ibid., 38.

12. Debruin, *Women and Health Research*, Vol. 2, 130.

13. Ibid.

14. L. Mitchell, quoted in *Women and Health Research*, Vol. 1, 80.

15. *Women and Health Research*, Vol. 1, 66.

16. Assessing Future Research Needs: Mental and Addictive Disorders in Women (Transcript), 221.

17. Ibid., 227.

18. Ibid., 228.

19. *Women and Health Research*, Vol. 1, 101.

20. Benet, *Women and Health Research*, Vol. 2, 42.

21. Ibid, 42-3.

22. *Women and Health Research*, Vol. 1, 29.

23. Weisman and Cassard, *Women and Health Research*, Vol. 2, 37-8.

24. Ibid., 37.

25. Polan, *Women and Health Research*, Vol. 2, 1.

26. Johnson and Fee, *Women and Health Research*, Vol. 2, 3.

27. Beecher, quoted in *Women and Health Research*, Vol. 1, 39.

28. *Women and Health Research*, Vol. 1, 40.

29. Johnson and Fee, *Women and Health Research*, Vol. 2, 3.

30. Ibid., 4.

31. Quoted in Johnson and Fee, *Women and Health Research*, Vol. 2, 5.

32. Johnson and Fee, *Women and Health Research*, Vol. 2, 1.

33. *Women and Health Research*, Vol. 1, 43-4.

34. *Opportunities for Research on Women's Health* (NIH 1992b), quoted in *Women and Health Research*, Vol. 1, 44.

35. *An Assessment of the NIH Women's Health Initiative*, 15.

36. Ibid., 90.

37. Ibid.
38. Ibid.
39. Ibid., 16.
40. *Women and Health Research*, Vol. 1, 109.
41. Ibid., 110.
42. Ibid.
43. Ibid., 111.
44. Johnson and Fee, *Women and Health Research*, Vol. 1, 5.
45. *Women and Health Research*, Vol. 1, 112.
46. Polan, *Women and Health Research*, Vol. 2, 1.
47. Sherwin, *Women and Health Research*, Vol. 2, 14.
48. DeBruin, *Women and Health Research*, Vol. 2, 136.
49. *Women and Health Research*, Vol. 1, 113.
50. Ibid., 99-100.
51. Ibid., 104.
52. Ibid., 100.
53. Ibid., 104-5.
54. Ibid.
55. *Strengthening Research in Academic OB/GYN Departments*, 75.
56. Ibid., 1.
57. Ibid., 7.
58. Ibid.
59. Ibid., 8.
60. Ibid., 83.
61. Ibid., 93.
62. Ibid., 101.
63. Polan, *Women and Health Research*, Vol. 2, 3.
64. *Developing New Contraceptives: Obstacles and Opportunities*, 85.
65. Ibid., 99-100.
66. Ibid., 4.
67. Ibid., 2.
68. *Strengthening Research,* 137.

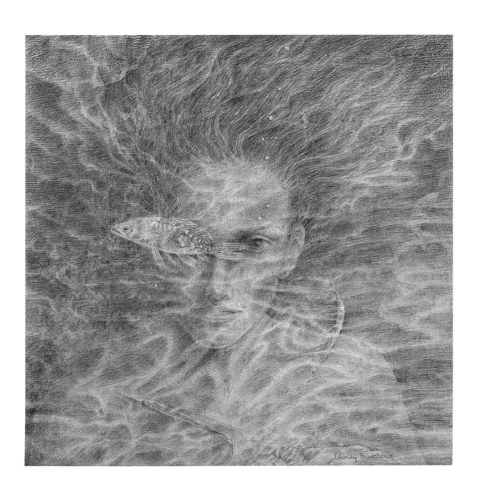

Wendy Fay Dixon
Deirdre (1982)
Silverpoint on paper
The National Museum of Women in the Arts
Gift of Deirdre Busenberg and the artist

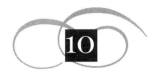

10

Looking Ahead

Within the memory of living Americans, there was a time when women generally spent the bulk of their years, and essentially their entire adult lives, bearing and nursing large numbers of children. Pregnancy happened outside of individual control but had the power to shape a person's identity, consciousness, and daily life. Death struck both young and old routinely, unpredictably, capriciously.

Today, the average American woman spends only 11% of the time between her menarche and her menopause—about 4 years—in active childbearing. Half have given birth to their last intended child by 30.[1] And the reproductive period, instead of consuming two-thirds of a lifetime as it formerly did, now typically accounts for well under a half. Many women now spend more years *after* their menopause than their foremothers spent as adults.

Few Americans now die in childbed or from infantile contagions. Sexually transmitted infections causing syphilis, gonorrhea, and cervical cancer no longer threaten certain death. No one need now sustain large numbers of closely spaced, undesired pregnancies or ransack her own body for the nutrients to feed an inexorably growing brood. American women who enjoy normal health and take reasonable care of it can now look forward to options and opportunities their grandmothers or great-grandmothers could not even have imagined.

Almost 60 years of active adulthood beckon today's healthy young girl. Indeed, the major ills that women face today arise in large part from the drastic reshaping of female lives that medical science has made possible within a current octogenarian's lifetime. We now live long enough to succumb to osteoporosis and Alzheimer's. We delay childbearing long enough to raise our risk of breast cancer. We eat richly enough to encourage cancers and cardiovascular disease. The current "epidemics" of the later years are, in a sense, the price we pay for the longer lives that most women now have the chance to live.

Despite this unprecedented progress, however, a lifetime of good health is, for far too many American women, nothing more than a "chance" that passes them by. A badly distorted health care system denies simple preventive care to countless people, but meanwhile almost indiscriminately provides vastly expensive therapies to repair predictable disasters. We transplant bone marrow in the terminal stages of breast cancer but bar the modestly priced mammograms that could have caught the disease early. We heroically rescue tiny infants with months of intensive care but withhold the simple prenatal care that might have assured them safe and timely delivery. We perform hundreds of thousands of abortions on young girls each year but block their access to the cheap contraceptives that would have prevented their pregnancies in the first place.

The research community, furthermore, fails to give adequate attention to issues vitally affecting female health. What can be done to lessen the painful and damaging social pressures that threaten the futures of so many adolescents? How can we organize care that helps the elderly preserve their dignity? Why can't we face the issues of sexuality frankly and openly enough to stem the spread of AIDS? How can we move forward in the search for more useful contraceptives? When will the ailments and experiences characteristic of women move out of the medical and scientific ghetto in which they have long languished and into the mainstream of thought and practice?

The women who will see the year 2000 have lived through a period of truly millennial change. They may well live to see other changes equally as great—perhaps now inconceivable lengthening of the life span, perhaps unimaginable control over fertility, perhaps the conquest of currently common diseases. Or they may witness, on the other hand, the uncontrollable rampage of HIV, or the ineluctable fall of more and more uninsured or inadequately insured Americans into medical penury and despair, or a rising tide of violence that will critically deform our society. Just as the lives we live today were beyond the dreams of our ancestors, so the lives our descendants will live may well be beyond ours.

What will not change, however, are the three forces that have shaped both this book and every female life: the interlocking pressures of physiology, gender, and social role. Women will continue to face particular physical and health challenges. Those challenges will differ from the ones faced by men. And the life demands and experiences that women encounter will continue to shape their responses.

As our nation's consciousness of women's health issues continues to rise, as women themselves take greater responsibility for their well-being and make greater demands on society for redress, and as more and more women gain positions of influence in the health professions, our health care system and the research enterprise that underlies it may respond increasingly effectively to these realities of female life. Or, bound in outdated biases and organizational principles, they may not. The outcome will depend on American women's ability to understand the issues that affect their health and then see that society responds.

IN CONCLUSION

This book represents many months spent pondering the changes of this century and immersed in the scrupulous research data assembled by IOM committee, conference, and staff members. Perhaps author's prerogative will permit it to end with what those excellent scientists would doubtlessly call a pair of anecdotal observations.

My paternal grandmother, Esther Malka Pomerantz Lieff, born in the 1880s, died of cervical or uterine cancer long before I could know her and well before anyone knew of the lifesaving power of the Pap smear. More than 50 years later, that simple test warned my gynecologist that her granddaughter needed a hysterectomy to escape her fate.

My maternal grandmother, Sarah Florin Jacobs, born in the

1890s, was stricken by blinding abdominal pain while preparing dinner for my grandfather in her seventy-ninth year. She died of a ruptured gallbladder the next day. In the quarter century that I knew her, she never once bestowed a gift without saying to the recipient, as I now wish for the reader, "May you use it in good health."

NOTE

1. Forrest (1991), 5.

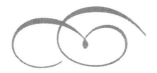

References

Unless otherwise noted, the Institute of Medicine publications that follow were published by the National Academy Press in Washington, D.C.

Access to Health Care in America, 1993. Michael Millman, ed.
AIDS and Behavior: An Integrated Approach, 1994. Judith D. Auerbach, Christina Wypijewska, and H. Keith H. Brodie, eds.
Allied Health Services: Avoiding Crises, 1988.
America's Aging: Health in an Older Society, 1985.
An Assessment of the NIH Women's Health Initiative, 1993. Susan Thaul and Dana Hotra, eds.
Assessing Future Research Needs: Mental and Addictive Disorders in Women. Summary of an Institute of Medicine Conference. 1991.
Assessing Future Research Needs: Mental and Addictive Disorders in Women. Unpublished transcript of a conference held on May 30-31, 1991.
Bereavement: Reactions, Consequences, and Care, 1984. Marian Osterweis, Fredric Solomon, and Morris Green, eds.
Body Composition and Physical Performance: Applications for the Military Services, 1992. Bernadette M. Marriott and Judith Grumstrup-Scott, eds.
Broadening the Base of Treatment for Alcohol Problems, 1990.
Clinical Applications of Mifepristone (RU 486) and Other Antiprogestins: Assessing the Science and Recommending a Research Agenda, 1993. Molla S. Donaldson, Laneta Dorflinger, Sarah S. Brown, and Leslie Z. Benet, eds.
Developing New Contraceptives: Obstacles and Opportunities, 1990.
Disability in America: Toward a National Agenda for Prevention, 1991. Andrew M. Pope and Alvin R. Tarlov, eds.
Eat for Life: The Food and Nutrition Board's Guide to Reducing Your Risk of Chronic Disease, 1992. Catherine E. Woteki and Paul R. Thomas, eds.
Effectiveness and Outcomes in Health Care, 1990. Kim A. Heithoff and Kathleen N. Lohr, eds.

Growing Up Tobacco Free: Preventing Nicotine Addiction in Children and Youths, 1994. Barbara S. Lynch and Richard J. Bonnie, eds.

Health and Behavior: Frontiers of Research in the Biobehavioral Sciences, 1982. David A. Hamburg, Glen R. Elliott, and Delores L. Parron, eds.

Healthy People 2000: Citizens Chart the Course, 1990. Michael A. Stoto, Ruth Behrens, and Connie Rosemont, eds.

In Her Lifetime: Female Morbidity and Mortality in Sub-Saharan Africa, 1996. Christopher P. Howson, Polly F. Harrison, Dana Hotra, and Maureen Law, eds.

Medical Professional Liability and the Delivery of Obstetrical Care. Volume I: Report of a Study, 1989.

Medical Professional Liability and the Delivery of Obstetrical Care. Volume II: An Interdisciplinary Review, 1989. Victoria P. Rostow and Roger J. Bulger, eds.

Medicare: A Strategy for Quality Assurance. Volume I: Report of a Study, 1990. Kathleen N. Lohr, ed.

Medicare: A Strategy for Quality Assurance. Volume II: Sources and Methods, 1990. Kathleen N. Lohr, ed.

Nutrition During Lactation, 1991.

Nutrition During Pregnancy: Weight Gain and Nutrient Supplements, 1990.

Proceedings of the 1992 IOM Annual Meeting. Unpublished transcript.

Reducing Risks for Mental Disorders: Frontiers for Preventive Intervention Research, 1994. Patricia J. Mrazek and Robert J. Haggerty, eds.

Research on Children and Adolescents with Mental, Behavioral, and Developmental Disorders: Mobilizing a National Initiative, 1989.

Science and Babies: Private Decisions, Public Dilemmas, 1990. By Suzanne Wymelenberg for the Institute of Medicine.

The Second Fifty Years: Promoting Health and Preventing Disability, 1992. Robert L. Berg and Joseph S. Cassells, eds.

Strengthening Research in Academic OB/GYN Departments, 1992. Jessica Townsend, ed.

Toward a National Health Care Survey: A Data System for the 21st Century, 1992. Gooloo S. Wunderlich, ed.

Toxic Shock Syndrome: An Assessment of Current Information and Future Research Needs, 1982.

Weighing the Options: Criteria for Evaluating Weight-Management Programs, 1995. Paul R. Thomas, ed.

Women and Health Research: Ethical and Legal Issues of Including Women in Clinical Trials. Volume 1: Report of a Study, 1994. Anna C. Mastroianni, Ruth Faden, and Daniel Federman, eds.

Women and Health Research: Ethical and Legal Issues of Including Women in Clinical Trials. Volume 2: Workshop and Commissioned Papers, 1994. Anna C. Mastroianni, Ruth Faden, and Daniel Federman, eds.

ADDITIONAL REFERENCES

Barrett-Connor, E. Epidemiology of Nutrition and Chronic Diseases in Women. Presentation at an IOM Symposium on Nutrition, Women, and Their Health, December 11, 1991.

Forrest, J. D. Socioeconomic and Demographic Trends Affecting Women's Health in the United States. Presentation at an IOM Symposium on Nutrition, Women, and Their Health, December 11, 1991.

Fridlund, K. E., King, N., and Askew, E. W. Nutrition Issues Unique to Women in the Army. Presentation at an IOM Symposium on Nutrition, Women, and Their Health, December 11, 1991.

King, J. C. Nutrition During Pregnancy and Lactation. Presentation at an IOM Symposium on Nutrition, Women, and Their Health, December 11, 1991.

Rasmussen, K. M. Effects of Pregnancy and Lactation on Women's Nutritional Status and Health. Presentation at an IOM Symposium on Nutrition, Women, and Their Health, December 11, 1991.

Rosenberg, I. Nutrition and Older Women. Presentation at an IOM Symposium on Nutrition, Women, and Their Health, December 11, 1991.

Scrimshaw, S. C. M. Social and Cultural Context for Women and Nutrition in Developing Countries. Presentation at an IOM Symposium on Nutrition, Women, and Their Health, December 11, 1991.

Stern, J. Dieting Behaviors and Weight-Maintenance Strategies Among Women. Presentation at an IOM Symposium on Nutrition, Women, and Their Health, December 11, 1991.

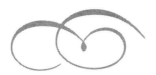

Index